Nursing the Dying Patient

Nursing the Dying Patient

Learning Processes for Interaction

Charlotte Epstein
Temple University

Reston Publishing Company, Inc., Reston, Virginia 22090
A Prentice-Hall Company

Library of Congress Cataloging in Publication Data

Epstein, Charlotte.
  Nursing the dying patient.

  Includes index.
  1. Terminal care. 2. Nurse and patient. 3. Med-
ical personnel and patient. 4. Role playing.
I. Title. [DNLM: 1. Death. 2. Nurse-patient
relations. 3. Terminal care. WY87 E65n]
R726.8.E67   610.73'6   74-34174
ISBN 0-87909-559-8
ISBN 0-87909-558-X pbk.

© 1975 by
Charlotte Epstein

10 9 8 7 6 5 4 3 2

Printed in the United States of America

. . . for all of us

Contents

Preface

Over and over again—in literature and in the clinical situation—dying patients say about themselves, "You still want to be a person." (Kübler-Ross) ". . . I can be a human being again." (Quint) "I'm not a dying patient; I'm a living person." (said to author.) It seems to me that, with these words, dying people are protesting an enormous injustice being done to them by those who have not been compelled to contemplate their own deaths.

Stereotyping is not a new problem in our society. We have a strong tendency to see people in terms of some arbitrary trait, such as skin color or religion, thus atributing to them a complex of behaviors and attitudes that are more misconception than fact. The almost impassable obstacle in recognizing the real person is our reluctance to make contact on any kind of equal status basis. Thus, white people avoid interacting with Black people because they fear, hate, or look down on them. Men are often reluctant to have women as colleagues in business. Black people might attribute to Puerto Rican people the same denigrating traits whites often attribute to Blacks.

In a curiously similar way, many of us seem to strip dying people of the traits that have identified them throughout their lives. The description, "dying," causes all other facets of the individual's personality to fade, and our behavior toward him becomes almost solely a function of his dying; that is, the behavior is *caused* by the dying—it is tailored for a dying, rather than for a living person.

xii   PREFACE

A demeaning attitude of others toward the patient seems to be the rule.
No matter how adequately the patient has functioned throughout his life,
the hospital society seems to assume that he is not competent to make
decisions governing his own life. Staff members may talk about him in his
presence as if he were insensate. The patient is often handled as if he has
lost all feelings of modesty and ability to reason. Not even his pain is given
respectful recognition; he is said to be "experiencing discomfort," an outrageous euphemism calculated to infuriate anyone suffering from pain.

Family members also stereotype the patient by divesting him of much
of his individuality. The healthy person sees the dying person as *finished.*
His life, except for his feelings of grief, loss and pain, is over. His hopes,
his desires, his pride and accomplishments are no longer considered in
interacting with him—though they may be talked *about* to other people,
in a sort of premature eulogizing. He is not even given credit for wanting
to know what is happening to him. Decisions about him are made without
consulting him, and *other people* decide that he should not be told that
he is dying.

To face a dying person is to be reminded of one's own mortality. Because the predominant emotion of the healthy toward the dying is fear,
avoidance becomes the operative behavior and interaction is only minimally productive.

Kastenbaum and Aisenberg *(The Psychology of Death)* believe that we
"out-group" the dying person, that "we shrink from the prospect of intimate contact with a dying person." They do not claim to know exactly
why this is so, but they feel a major reason for our avoidance is that "we
do not know what to do when we are with a dying person. Nobody has
given us adequate instruction. We do not like to find ourselves in a
situation—especially an important situation—for which we lack . . . responses."

There is probably little relationship between what people think they
feel about death and what they actually feel when death must be faced.
Listening to lectures about death and dying seem to influence what students think they think about death. In such a setting, there is little opportunity to examine one's own possible behavior toward dying people. It
would seem more useful (1) to help students become aware of their own
behaviors, (2) to examine patient behaviors, and (3) to examine and
practice alternative behaviors. Students should—in simulated situations—
actually behave sometimes like a patient and other times like a nurse.
The objective of this role-playing is to arrive at a repertory of behaviors
that will be helpful to the person in the interactive situation who needs
help.

It may seem obvious that when the dying patient and the nurse come
together, it is the patient who most needs the help. However, from what
we are learning of such interactions, it is not unusual for the professional

to be most in need of help. There have even been times when the patient has recognized this need and tried to provide for it by expressing sympathy, or has demonstrated empathy by avoiding talk of death.

Perhaps in the process of developing awareness and practicing alternative responses, each nurse will find links to other people who are struggling to make this aspect of their professional life more productive and satisfying.

An explanatory note

People who use this book will discover that it does not always make a distinction between teachers and students. It seems to speak alternately to the teacher and to the students. The blurring of the traditional dividing line between the two is intentional. In our attempts to learn how to face our own dying and how to interact effectively with dying people, we are all teachers. In each situation, whether in the classroom, in the professional meeting, or in the hospital room, the teacher of the moment is that person who has the insight, sensitivity, and skill that are needed at that moment. If the teaching directions in an exercise seem to speak to someone, then let him take on the leadership role, even though he is not the teacher of record. There is nothing to prevent him from participating as a student in the next exercise if someone else feels comfortable as the teacher in this exercise.

The alternation between teacher role and student role relieves any one person of the whole burden of leadership in this difficult area of learning, and may help more people risk becoming involved in a subject about which all of us know so little.

CHARLOTTE EPSTEIN

Heightening Self-awareness

chapter one

---◄◄►►---

The Learning Process

In the classroom or on the job

Most of the recent writing about death and dying has been descriptive.
The dying process has been observed and recorded; the behavior of nurses
and other medical personnel has been described; and the responses of
bereaved families have become a part of the contemporary data that help
to fill the gap in our knowledge about dying.

With characteristic enthusiasm about the efficacy of amassing information, teachers of those who treat the dying use new data the way teachers
use most data: they insist that students "learn" it, and they test them
to be sure that they are learning it. Theoretically, the wealth of information is supposed to improve the nurse's ability to treat dying people. It
should increase the student's sensitivity and develop his or her skill. The
information is supposed to overcome strong tendencies in a person to
avoid the subject of death and give reassurance that those who talk
about death are not neurotically morbid.

However, like information about other subjects, it is only the *beginning* of wisdom and skills. Before students and health personnel can use
the available information, a connection must be made between that
information and the interactive situation between personnel and dying
patient. That link can be fashioned only out of involvement in processes
that help the student anticipate his own reactions and the reactions of

others: processes that insure the development of a repertory of alternative responses and solutions to problems, so that the student may have
something to choose from when he is faced with the real situation. These
processes should provide him an opportunity to contemplate his own
death and come to terms with some of the feelings that contemplation
inevitably invokes. Even though we now have a rapidly growing body of
descriptive data that is at last emerging from its cover of fear and sentimentality, it simply is not fair, either to the student or the dying patient,
to expect their interaction to begin with only a background of required
reading.

This book was not designed to provide answers to all the problems
associated with treating the dying. Many answers have not yet been discovered, and most answers are to be found—as in most human interaction
—only by the participants themselves. However, the learning situations
described here provide opportunity for discovering some of those answers.

The exercises in this book cannot take the place of interacting with
someone who is dying. At some point in the development of awareness,
sensitivity, skill—and even in the acquisition of knowledge—we must
become involved in the real-life situation. However, involvement in the
exercises should make that first professional contact a more comfortable
one, and subsequent interaction more productive.

There are skills involved in interacting effectively with dying people,
just as there are skills needed in other human interactions. And skills
are for learning. One may start the learning on the job—making all the
trials and errors that were made by people before him. The danger is that
the employee, discouraged and intimidated by his errors and his feelings
of inadequacy, may give up and go on to other kinds of work. (This says
nothing, of course, about the unfairness to patients who are the victims
of repetitious errors each time new people come on the job. Caring for
people is not quite the same as punching out metal discs. Errors hurt!)

Must we forget all we know about education just because we are suddenly aware of the need to learn a new set of skills? No, the fact is, we
can begin our learning in the classroom, and thus be better prepared
when we come into contact with dying people. Unfortunately, the new
practitioners in the care of the dying have generally not been trained in
education, so their approach to preparing other practitioners does not
draw on the philosophies and strategies of teaching. Though the two or
three well-known names in the field are obviously—as their successes
attest—natural teachers, there is little evidence that their successes can
be replicated in most medical treatment facilities. The available natural
teachers are too few to reach all the people who need to learn how to
interact effectively with dying patients.

Our alternative then, should be to apply our knowledge of teaching other subjects to teach people to interact effectively with those who are dying. And that means starting the learning in a classroom setting.

Dr. Cicely Saunders of St. Christopher's Hospice in London recently replied, in answer to a question, that the best way to learn to live is to go about the business of living. She suggested that people trying to learn to treat the dying find the dying person down the street, or the bereaved family around the corner and interact with them. (Learning by doing— or by *living*.) However, it is not helpful to hundreds of nursing students and medical students who are thrust into hospitals with no preparation for treating those who are dying to exhort them to learn by *living*. A few hours of simulation training or skill practice may be more useful in helping them avoid mistakes and trauma, guilt and self-doubt.

Developing self-awareness

You do not learn the really important things about interacting with dying people from secondhand information. In the final analysis, it is what you find in yourself that makes any human interaction you have more effective and more satisfying.

Nevertheless, the information that others cull from their experiences with dying people is valuable. It gives the inexperienced some signposts so that they do not enter into every new relationship making the same old mistakes. For example, experienced observers note that a conspiracy to keep a patient from the knowledge of his imminent death is a conspiracy doomed to failure; the patient can usually detect from the changes in the behavior of the people around him and from the nature of their responses to his questions that he is going to die. Thus the inexperienced person can use this information to resist the temptation to engage in such a conspiracy of silence.

Similarly, peers and supervisors, as well as experimental evidence, can inform the nurse that people literally do keep a greater distance between themselves and the dying patient than they do between themselves and the patient with a favorable prognosis. But the nurse must go beyond this information to recognize that tendency in herself, to examine the sources of her own discomfort, and she must ultimately make a conscious effort to change her own behavior if she is to be effective in providing care for the dying patient.

Thinking about one's own death

It is not easy for a healthy person to think seriously of his own dying. It would seem, however, that we must do this in order to come to terms with our deep-seated feelings about death and then learn to interact productively with people who are dying. If we run from our own feelings and are afraid to admit them, then we will surely run from the dying, afraid to face them and the feelings they can no longer deny.

Consequently, much of the preparation we must make before we undertake the treatment of dying patients involves learning to face the reality of our own death. Perhaps in some muted and less profound way, we can go through a simulation of the dying process that Kübler-Ross describes *(On Death and Dying)* and so perceive—if only dimly—something of what the dying person is experiencing.

We, of course, are not compelled to confront immediately the information that our death is imminent. The odds are that we have more time. Therefore, we can start with a more oblique look at the topic and then work more gradually around to the heart of the matter.

chapter two

————◆◄◆►◆————

Exercises for
Developing Self-awareness

Where Do I Stand?

Consider this question: How do you want other people to act when you die?

Most people do not appear to have much trouble responding to this question. They seem able to answer it—often in an offhand way—and then quickly drop the subject, as if it made no great impression on them. It seems to be fruitful to use such a familiar question to encourage students to respond. If they are urged to stay with the topic for a while, they may begin to consider it more seriously.

To help people see the many possible points of view, draw a continuum of responses on the chalkboard, making the line between the two extremes quite long. (Use a whole wall if it is available, or get 15 or 20 feet of wrapping paper and tape it on a wall.)

I just want my body disposed of in the most efficient way, with no mention made of me after I'm dead.	I want my family to mourn me every day of their lives— unconsolable in their grief.

As opinions are expressed, people could decide where they belonged on the continuum. They could even be encouraged to go to the board and write in their own point of view in the appropriate place.

Discussion

Students have commented upon this exercise in a variety of ways:

"I never really thought about it before."

"I know people don't like to talk about such things. I don't even like to think about such things."

"I never knew people felt all these different ways."

"I don't know *what* I really want now. I'll have to think about it some more."

"I never really knew that this was the way I felt. It sort of makes me think that maybe I'm not as unselfish as I like to think I am."

"I always knew I loved my family. But I didn't realize I wanted them to be so broken up about me."

What do I really want from the people I love?

This exercise explores more of our expectations concerning the people closest to us. It seems, indirectly, to offer clues to how *we* would like to be treated should we learn that we are dying. If we are fairly clear concerning expectations about our own deaths, it may be easier to avoid confusing our own needs and desires with the patients' needs—thinking we are doing what the patient wants, when we are really doing what *we* would want were we in the patient's place.

Work in groups of about 10 people, giving yourself enough space so that you can move about during role playing. On a sheet of paper, write the name of one person who is important to you—your mother, your best friend, your husband, wife, colleague. Imagine that this person has just been told that you are going to die very soon. Write a description of the way you would want this person to react to the news of your imminent death.

When everyone has finished, put the paper away. Now read the following:

You have just had a shocking experience. During a routine examination a virtually fatal tumor is discovered in a spot that rules out the feasibility of surgery. Though your family physician is gentle, he makes it clear that your prognosis is not favorable. He offers to break the news to the person important to you, and you agree to let him do so.

Sit for a moment and think about all this, trying to feel the sense of shock that fills you.

Now, one person in the group can take the role of the physician and another the role of your own important person. Role play the scene of the physician telling this person about your imminent death.

When the scene is over, let the observers tell you what you said and what feelings you revealed when you were told the news.

Afterwards, read from your paper what *you* said about how you wanted that person to respond to the knowledge of your dying. Was there a difference between what you wrote and the way you role-played that person? If there was, how do you account for the difference? Can others in the group help you account for the difference? If there was no difference, is it because you know your loved one very well and are able to closely duplicate his behavior? Or is it that you are acting the way you *hope* he will respond?

You might ask yourself these questions:

1. Am I saying I want one thing from the people I love, but in reality want something quite different?
2. Do I want from the people I love something I don't really expect to get?
3. Am I really dissatisfied with my own reactions, wishing that *I* would behave differently?

After other people have taken their turns in this role playing, discuss these questions:

1. Generally, what has been revealed about expected behavior and actual observed behavior?
2. Generally, how do people seem to feel about their own behavior in such a situation?
3. What new thoughts have occurred to you about your own dying?

Discussion

In one such role-playing, a doctor insisted that he wanted his wife to finish her grieving quickly and then go on with her life as before. He acted out this behavior by his initial shock, a few tears, a deep breath, and that was it. When the observers in his group protested that his behavior didn't seem real, he finally confessed that he didn't really want his wife to be so calm about his death. He was actually *afraid* that she would behave this way because she was a self-centered person who cared more for herself than others.

As the discussion continued, he cautiously admitted that he wanted his wife and children to "really be sorry" about his dying and to show it. On past occasions when families had taken a prognosis of death calmly, he had thought it cold and inappropriate, and had resented their "selfishness." Was it possible, he finally asked himself, that his own needs prevented patients and families from reaching a level of calm acceptance of death?

A physiotherapist was unable to act out the screaming, uncontrollable behavior she believed her mother would demonstrate. As she described this behavior to her observers, it became clear that screaming and crying frightened and embarrassed her. Her impulse was to run from it; and the few times she had encountered such behavior professionally, she had done just that.

The members of her group tried to help her understand the need for some people to express their feelings freely and the value of such outpouring of grief to the final resolution of the grieving process. As the course developed, and her experience with talking about dying increased, she learned to cry—and to accept comfort.

Talking about our own deaths

Sooner or later we come to the point where we must begin to talk about our own deaths. Such an emotion-laden subject is best handled in a small group. The small group encourages a feeling of intimacy that is necessary for revealing what, perhaps, has never been revealed before. It is easier, also, to estimate the trustworthiness of a small number of people, and so feel freer to risk talking about our private feelings, less fearful that this knowledge will be used against us. No "leader" is needed in such a group; contributions will be spontaneous and will depend on how quickly the group members feel comfortable with each other. Certainly no one should take notes of what is said or attempt to report the "proceedings" to a larger group. There should be an expectation of reasonable confidentiality. After all, the group members are using each other as sounding-boards so that they may better understand *themselves*. What would be the point of repeating what is said to people who are not a part of the process?

Form groups of about eight students, sitting close together so that, even though they are in a room with other students, they can talk to each other quietly with a certain amount of privacy. (When the group is larger than eight people, it will be more difficult to keep voices low and still be heard by everyone in the group.)

Before the discussion begins, sit quietly for a few minutes and think about your own death. Say nothing. Wrap yourself around the thought of your own dying. Let the feelings come. Now, try to tell each other how you feel. Never mind how you think you *ought* to feel, what a "professional" *should feel*. Your feelings are real, and you have a right to them. Other people have no business evaluating your feelings or telling you that you shouldn't feel that way. If the members of your group listen to and accept each other's feelings, you will feel more and more comfortable about sharing them with each other.

How can you make it clear to your colleagues that you *do* accept how they feel? Do you evaluate when you think you are comforting? Do you try to impose your point of view on others when you think you are listening? Are you giving a lecture when you think you are having a conversation?

Following is a partial transcript of a discussion about dying among students of nursing and their classroom instructor. Don't look at the key to the numbered comments until you have tried to determine for yourself what the speaker is really saying.

(There is a period of silence that seems to stretch endlessly, though actually it lasts for only about three minutes. Finally Ms. A makes a sound of impatience.)

Ms. A: This is ridiculous!

(Silence.)

Ms. A: (Defiantly) There's no point talking about this! It's just silly!

Ms. B: It's not silly.[1]

Ms. C: I'm only 21 years old! I can't possibly imagine dying!

Ms. A: That's what I mean! There's no point to it.

Ms. B: You're just avoiding it.[2] Nobody likes to think about it.

Mr. D: I'll probably die of cancer.

Ms. A: (Almost angrily) What makes you say a thing like that?

Mr. D: (Very matter-of-factly) Most of the people in my family—on both sides—died of cancer. So naturally, I assume I probably will get cancer at some point in my life!

Ms. A: That's stupid! [3]

Mr. D: What are you getting so mad about? You'd think I was saying you're going to die of cancer.

Ms. A: Aaaaa! (Indicating dismissal)

Ms. B: It could happen to any one of us. It's not pleasant to think about.

Ms. E: I'd rather be dead than incapacitated. If I can't respond to my environment, I might as well be dead already.

Ms. F: That's terrible.[4] I don't feel that way at all. As long as I had peace of mind in my last few days, I wouldn't mind dying all that much.

Ms. E: How can you have peace of mind if you know that you'll be dead in a few days?!

Ms. G: None of this is real! You're not saying what you're really feeling![5]

Ms. A: How do *you* know what we feel? Why don't you talk about your own feelings?

Ms. F: I hope I don't die before I've really had a chance to live.

Ms. G: (In a low voice) It's terrible to think of yourself dying.

   (Silence.)

Ms. A: (Giggle) It frightens me to death.

Mr. D: (In a low voice) I watched my father die of cancer. I saw him waste away to 75 pounds.

Ms. A: Did he know he was dying?

Ms. E: I want to die quickly—no long, drawn-out thing. I'd permit as little medical intervention as possible, once I knew I was dying.

Ms. H: You know what really frightens me about dying? Because I don't know what will happen to my soul, and that's something no one can tell me.

Ms. A: I'm just scared of the pain. The pain. . . .

Mr. D: Nobody wants pain.[6]

Ms. G: Why does it frighten me so much? What am I really afraid of?

Mr. D: You really don't have to be afraid. There are stages of dying that everyone goes through: denial, rage, grieving, and acceptance. When you finally accept that you're going to die, you're not afraid any more. The experts say. . . .[7]

Ms. A: I don't care what the experts say. I just know how I feel.

Ms. B: Let's talk about living. After all, our job is to heal.

Discussion Key

[1] Ms. B is telling Ms. A that her feelings—whatever they are—are not to be seriously considered. Ms. B might do better to try to discover what Ms. A's feelings really are beneath her frantic attempt to avoid the topic.

[2] Ms. B is more intent on disagreeing with Ms. A than in encouraging her to say more.

[3] Here Ms. A is doing to Mr. D what has been done to her by Ms. B.

[4] Why can't Ms. F just say how she feels? Why must she first put a value on Ms. E's feeling?

[5] This accusation leads to an argument. Maybe if Ms. G expressed her own feelings a little more directly, the others would too.

[6] This is platitude. It reduces the importance of what Ms. A is saying. Mr. D is implying that, since everyone knows that nobody wants pain, there's no point in hearing Ms. A say she's frightened of pain.

[7] Mr. D is giving a lecture on dying, again denying the significance of everyone else's feelings (and, incidentally, avoiding expressing his own.)

Do I really believe I am going to die?

Complete the following questionnaire, first answering the question, "Do you really believe you are going to die?" (Yes or no.) Check *Agree* or *Disagree* for each of the following statements as it applies to you:

	Agree	*Disagree*
1. When I read statistics of traffic deaths, I think it unlikely that such a thing can happen to me.	_____	_____
2. I have never had someone close to me—*of my own age*—die.	_____	_____
3. I think that my death will be only a temporary separation from those I love.	_____	_____
4. Inside I really believe that the secret of eternal life will one day be discovered.	_____	_____
5. I don't think much about death.	_____	_____
6. Of course I know that all living things die. But if I take care of myself and avoid foolish risks there's no reason to think about dying for a long, long time.	_____	_____
7. Though war is hard, I think it can be a glorious experience—for a man and for a nation.	_____	_____
8. I think when a relatively young person gets sick and dies, there must have been something in his attitude and approach to life that made him susceptible to the disease; that is, he really *wanted* to die.	_____	_____
9. I read the newspaper or listen to the news fairly often.	_____	_____
10. It is impossible for anyone to accept the knowledge of his own death peacefully.	_____	_____
11. No one has a right to decide that at some arbitrary point it is useless to continue medical treatment.	_____	_____

Discussion

This is not a scientifically validated or even orthodox attitude questionnaire with results that can be compiled, and generalizations that can be made about people's belief in their own mortality. However, as you consider each statement you may get some clues about the depth and intensity of your own need to negate the reality of death.

ITEMS 1, 5, 9: When a person says he does not think much about death —especially when he is young and in good health, and has no day-to-day contact with people who are dying—it does not necessarily indicate that he is denying the reality of his own death. However, when one looks at other facets of our culture, one must conclude that *not* thinking about death requires some active process of repression. The daily media accounts are full of traffic accidents that take a frightening toll of life every day. To ignore the possibility that we may very well become part of the statistics is behavior that seems to have a large denial component. Every day of our lives we walk on sidewalks, cross the streets, ride as passengers, and drive our cars, and each behavior carries greater risk that we will become victims of a traffic accident. Many of the "horror" advertisements of safety organizations also make us realize that the possibility of our death is ever-present. Not to think about death in such circumstances must mean that we are, as a nation, engaged in an unconscious conspiracy to deny our own deaths.

ITEM 7: The newspapers also give graphic evidence of the high incidence of death from war and accidents, but many of us believe that war is patriotic, adventuresome, and even glorious, and that accidents always happen to someone else. Of course, some newspaper stories about war aid in the process of denial, making the killing and the dying out to be a bloodless duel of honor.

ITEM 2: One of the experiences that seems to halt the persistence of denial concerning our own death is having someone die who is important to us and near our own age. If a good friend, or a close cousin, or a sister two years younger has died, the myth of our own immortality often dies too—or is, at least, somewhat more difficult to believe. Not thinking about dying, not talking or reading about it can keep awareness to a minimum.

ITEMS 3, 4: Statements 3 and 4 reveal a belief in death as only temporary. Admittedly, it is very difficult to imagine our own nonexistence. Perhaps it is impossible to do so. However, to admit this difficulty is quite different from believing in immortality or in continuation of life after death. The first statement (#3) recognizes an apparent limitation of human perception; the second ignores the limitation and arbitrarily adjusts the reality to suit the limited perception.

ITEMS 6, 8: The individual in item #6 believes that he can control the length of his life. This belief is an extension of the idea that a person controls his own destiny, consciously making choices that influence the course of his life. Just what measure of control any individual has over his life is discussed later more fully. However, the inescapable fact is, though we may successfully avoid some particular ways of dying, we cannot avoid *every* way. Item #8, particularly, sounds almost as if the speaker believes that, if he does not *want* to die, he *will* not die. The denial is evident.

ITEM 10: It would appear that the person who believes this statement is reflecting his own attitude about dying. We have evidence that people who are dying often do reach a condition of peace and acceptance. The person who rejects this information probably feels that *he* could never peacefully accept the knowledge of his own dying. He must feel, then, that the emotions surrounding death are all unpleasant ones—fear, anger, terror, anxiety. Since it is only natural to try to avoid such unpleasant feelings, it is just as natural to avoid the dying person, and avoid the thought of one's own death.

ITEM 11: To take such an adamant stand against any judgment that medical treatment will not save a person's life seems to be, in a subtle way, a denial of death. The implication is that life is always possible, that death is never inevitable. It is this kind of denial that, in some respects, makes a person insist that the machines be kept going despite evidence that the patient will never be able to function again.

Now that you have read the discussion of the questionnaire, how would you answer the question, "Do you really believe you are going to die?" Have you changed your answer? Have you learned something about yourself that you never knew before? Maybe you would be interested in sharing some of these new insights with your colleagues. If you would, be sure you do so in small groups rather than in a large class. Perhaps many of you would be reluctant to talk about your most significant insights in front of a large group.

How do I really feel about the patient who is dying?

Sooner or later you will be expected to treat a patient who is dying. What thoughts and feelings do you have as you think about this? Think about your *true* feelings, not what you think they *ought* to be. For now, try to forget all the things you have learned about how a "professional" must respond to a dying patient, how a "mature" adult must feel about death, and how your family feels about death and dying. To help you do this, complete the following attitude self-check. You need not reveal any of your answers to your colleagues or your instructor unless you choose to do so. Just put a check next to each statement that expresses how you feel.

_____ 1. I expect to feel very uncomfortable when I have to talk to a dying patient.
_____ 2. I wish I knew what to say to a patient who knows he is dying.
_____ 3. I wouldn't want to be the one to tell a patient he is dying.
_____ 4. At the point when there's nothing more medical science can do for a patient, then the responsibility of the doctor and nurse is only to make him as comfortable as possible physically.
_____ 5. I am frankly frightened at the thought of caring for a dying patient. I am afraid the patient will ask me if he is dying—or other questions about his condition—that I am not supposed to answer.
_____ 6. I think I can help make a patient more comfortable with the fact of his death.
_____ 7. I worry that I will get too fond of a dying patient and won't be able to control my feelings.
_____ 8. I can't imagine anyone ever being free of the fear of dying.
_____ 9. I don't think a person should be told he's dying. There's no point in adding to his suffering.
_____10. I think people are most afraid of death when they're about my age than at any other age.
_____11. I don't think death should be discussed in front of children.
_____12. I must admit to a feeling of disgust at the thought of being around a person who is dying.
_____13. Being around a dying person would just keep reminding me that I will also die.
_____14. I think people can wish you dead.
_____15. Being around someone who is sick or dying would make me feel proud of my good physical condition.

Discussion

When everyone has completed the attitude self-check, you may, as a group, decide to talk about some of the items that you found particularly interesting for one reason or another. Of course you may choose not to discuss this at all at this time—or even not to read the following comments:

1. Perhaps what is bothering you most is the thought of the first time you will have to talk to a patient who is dying. Maybe learning that other people share your anxiety will help you feel better about yourself—make you feel less guilty or "selfish" because you are thinking of your own feelings instead of the patient's.

2. If you are worried about what to say to a dying patient, afraid that you will not know what the "appropriate" words are, the exercises in this book should help to provide an opportunity for finding the words.

3. Perhaps, also, as you continue your involvement in the subject of dying, you will learn to let the patient take the lead in talking about his own dying. You may find that it is rarely necessary for you or anyone else to be the first to mention the word death.

4. You may also realize—as you never have before—that there is much you can do for a dying person beyond the purely medical-physical. In addition, it may gratify you to learn that there is much a dying person can do for you if you lend yourself to the relationship as a whole person, not just as a professional.

5. Some of the things you learn may be useful to the other people who work with you in caring for dying patients. Maybe you can explore some effective ways of communicating these things to them. If you are successful, the words "not supposed to" will disappear from the list of hospital rules.

6. You *know* you can!

7. If by control you mean hide your feelings, you may ultimately decide that a show of honest feeling is both useful and desirable—for you and the patient.

8. You may even come to terms with the inevitability of your own death and be able to express your honest feelings.

9. You will surely discover, in the course of your studying, that it is often a misconception to suppose that knowing you are dying causes more suffering than having the knowledge kept from you by an uneasy conspiracy among those who care about you.

10. Avoiding the topic may be more comfortable, but it can be only a temporary comfort. Facing the fear makes facing death easier.

11. Children are aware of death. They are more disturbed at the whispers and the way adults fall silent or change the subject when they come in than they would be if their feelings were permitted free expression.

12. There is an undercurrent in our culture that makes a connection

between dying and failure. The dying person's loss of control over his own life has ties—in subtle ways—to a personality defect of weakness and ineptitude. Intellectually, we can easily repudiate such nonsense, but the feeling may creep into our consciousness in spite of ourselves.

13. It is undoubtedly true that being with a dying person makes it more difficult for us to deny our own mortality.

14. This is another explanation of the guilt people feel when someone dies. Children, especially, may believe that their anger and even death wishes caused the death of a loved one. Perhaps some of this childhood belief remains to haunt us.

15. If there is a lingering idea that the person who is dying has someway brought it upon himself, it may account for the feeling of superiority of the healthy person. How shocking it must be for someone like this one day to be suddenly faced with the fact of his own imminent death!

The Stages of Dying

chapter three

Denial

The patient's behavior

It is not surprising that people find it difficult to accept the fact of their own dying. The self cannot seem to perceive its own nonexistence, and our culture reinforces this inability and even encourages it. Consequently, it is not difficult to identify the things people say and do that indicate their denial of death.

This is not to say that each patient proceeds neatly through the "stages of dying" as defined by Kübler-Ross, at each stage wearing a placard inscribed with "Denial," "Anger," etc. It means, rather, that from the time a fatal disease is diagnosed until the time the person dies, there are periods when the patient needs to deny that he is dying. Many patients go through a large interval of time near the beginning when they do most of the denying. Further intervals of denial involve somewhat shorter time spans. Some patients find it necessary to deny with some people and not with others. This is not a conscious pretense of the patient to protect a member of his family or a health-care person who obviously cannot handle dying, and may be caught up in a denial of his own. It is an unconsciously motivated behavior precipitated by the need to maintain a particular relationship.

Denial can be detected in the following words and actions:

21

1. The patient says, "No, I don't believe it."
2. The patient seeks treatment from a "healer" not authorized by medical authorities.
3. The patient attributes specific symptoms of his illness to other—less serious—medical conditions.
4. The patient goes from doctor to doctor searching for a more favorable diagnosis.
5. The patient does not understand the implications of his illness. He is like the man who attributed his cancer that necessitated removal of a kidney to a bump he gave his back when walking past a desk several months earlier.
6. The patient says he believes an error has been made on his tests or records.
7. The patient uses euphemisms to identify his illness, such as referring to an open, cancerous sore as a bad leg.
8. The patient temporarily forgets that he has knowledge of his dying.
9. The patient talks about and plans for the future as if she will still be alive.
10. The patient refuses follow-up treatment, indicating that the surgery or the initial crisis, once over, indicates she is well again.
11. The patient never talks about dying.
12. The patient asks no questions about his condition, even about the obvious symptoms.
13. The patient complains that no one will tell her what is wrong, though different staff members have repeatedly tried to make her understand.
14. The patient refuses treatment, preferring to let the symptoms "disappear" by themselves.
15. The patient actually denies the reason for his admission, insisting that he has been overworking or just needs a check-up.
16. The patient accepts treatment in the expressed belief that it will facilitate cure.
17. The patient does not recognize drastic changes in his physical appearance.
18. The patient talks about the stay in hospital as if it were for a very short period.
19. The patient expresses belief in a life after death that is very much like the life she now knows.
20. The patient knows what his illness is and what is happening to him, yet he rejects the belief that he will die.
21. The patient talks about her illness as if it were minor.

The practitioner's response

Essentially, the practitioner's problem is dealing with his own tendency to avoid confronting the fact of death. This can trap him into concurring with the patient's denial, reinforcing it, and actually preventing the patient from moving from denial to a more realistic stance. It is difficult to heed the admonition that the patient's denial must be accepted, and at the same time refrain from preventing the patient from relinquishing denial when he is able to do so. It is necessary to accept the patient's denial in such a way as to hold up to him a point of reference in reality. When he is able, he will then use the reference point to carry him to a more realistic view of his illness.

It is also difficult to distinguish between the patient's need for denial and our own need. For example, the nurse may actually precipitate the patient's denial by emitting such strong denial cues that the weaker reality cues offered by the rest of the staff are easily blocked from the patient's awareness.

Sometimes, the doctor may be unable to accept the fact that further medical treatment would not be useful. It takes a profound acceptance of death for a doctor to admit that it would be useless for a person in the last stages of metastatic carcinoma to be treated with vast dosages of antibiotics when she contracts pneumonia. Such measures may force a patient into clinging to denial of his dying, in the face of everything she has been told about her primary illness.

Denial by the patient's family

Besides accepting the patient's denial and maintaining a reality reference for him, the practitioner should provide him with experiences to help relieve his feelings of panic and reduce his feelings of stress. The obvious nursing/medical services to make the patient physically comfortable need no elaboration here. The need for other kinds of services are not so often recognized. Often the patient needs support in dealing with the denial of his family and friends. The nurse may let the patient practice on her what he might say to a member of his family. Or she may offer to act as a temporary liaison to his family, carrying the message to them that the patient realizes the fact of his death and that their continued denial would only serve to isolate him. Unable to talk to them about what is uppermost in his mind, he will be forced to pretend interest in other matters or keep silent. Either choice would have the effect of putting up a wall between them, thus leaving the patient deprived of the comfort of those he loves.

Exercises for Skill Development

1. Practicing denial

To summarize: Dr. Kübler-Ross has observed that most patients upon learning they have a terminal illness first react by denying the fact. The patients often talk about errors in diagnosis, discuss their illness as if it were minor, and make plans for the future. The doctors, nurses, and family members may also engage in this denial and thus delay the time when the patient accepts death with a certain amount of peace.

It might be useful for us, while we are healthy and in the relatively safe environment of the classroom, to look more closely at behaviors that indicate denial and to get some idea of how it feels to use them and to see them.

Pair up with another member of your group and go to a corner where you can have some privacy. One of you should assume the role of doctor, the other of patient. Now, the doctor comes into the patient's room and says, "I'm sorry, but the tumor was malignant." The patient responds with some kind of denial: (1) he may seem to have misunderstood the diagnosis; (2) he may refuse to accept the diagnosis as true; (3) he may ignore the diagnosis; (4) he may physically run from the diagnosis.

Pick one of these manifestations of denial and act out the scene. Afterwards, switch roles and repeat the activity, again permitting the patient a choice in the kind of denial he manifests.

Try, as you play the roles, to be the patient who has just been told—in effect—that he is dying. (In actuality, a diagnosis of malignancy does not inevitably mean death. The patient may merely think that cancer is equated with dying, and his behavior must be understood in these terms.) Amplify your initial response, making it clear just what form your denial is taking.

Let the doctor respond in any way he is moved to respond and carry the dialogue for as long as you wish.

When it is over, see if the doctor can identify the type of denial the patient demonstrated. Let the patient explain how he felt about the doctor's responses, and whether or not he thought they were helpful. Discuss how the denial of death made you feel, as the patient and as the doctor.

Discussion of the Exercise

What are some of the things you might say and do as the patient in relation to this exercise?

1. The patient who seems to misunderstand the diagnosis may respond to the doctor's words by saying something like, "Oh, that's a relief! I was afraid I had something terrible" or "Are you sure it's nothing serious?" He may begin immediate preparations to leave the hospital so he can resume work or caring for the family.
2. Refusal to believe the diagnosis may take the form of saying, "No, that's impossible!" or "It can't happen to me!" or just an emphatic, "No! No!"
3. Some patients may ask, "Are you sure you have it right? Can't there be a mistake?" They may insist that the X-rays or lab reports were mixed up.
4. She may listen to the diagnosis and immediately begin to talk about something that has no relation to it; a recent visit from her husband, something a child told her on the phone, the pressures of her job.
5. He may merely begin to dress and say that he is going home.

As Kübler-Ross points out, often the doctor also needs to deny the fact of death; thus, he reinforces the patient's response and contributes to the prolongation of the denial stage. Although the patient needs a period of denial to give himself time to cope more realistically with dying, the doctor cannot afford such behavior. Though he must listen to his patient talk out his denial, and indicate clearly that he is available to listen and to help, he cannot—out of his own need to deny death—mislead the patient.

Consequently, the doctor should not say to the patient, "You'll be fine" or "Everything will be all right" or "That's right, it's nothing serious." Nor should he leave immediately after the patient's response. By remaining he may give the patient opportunity to give some sign of recognition of the truth even if it is only a momentary recognition.

Of course, it is not useful for the doctor to say to the denying patient, "What are you talking about? Didn't you hear me? I said you have cancer!" Although the doctor must not take the lead in denial or re-inforce the patient's denial, he must in his responses be guided by what the dying person needs at the time. There is nothing to be gained from forcing a person to admit he is dying when he is obviously not prepared to deal with such information. The chances are that his defenses will only be strengthened by such a demand and the period of his denial lengthened.

One of the most interesting experiences I had was in testing this exercise in denial with a group of people who had no connection with the health professions. As each person assumed the role of the dying patient, the ease and creativity with which he avoided the truth was startling. Not all role-playing situations are so skillfully managed—especially by people who have had little or no experience with such an activity. I can only conclude that the propensity for denial in this kind of situation is very great indeed.

Over and over again, many participants "misunderstood" the significance of the diagnosis. There were long monologues about tumors being easy to cut out, how many people they knew who had such "simple" operations. Their impression was that a tumor was somehow detached from surrounding organs and tissue, and needed only a minor incision to set it free.

Some role-players felt they were "immune" to tumors. Others asked, weren't tumors caused by viruses? Well, they just weren't susceptible to viruses; they never came down with anything like that. Some people told involved stories of experiences they had had with errors made in large institutions. A few recalled with great feeling and no small triumph outrageous errors that the University had made on their records last week, last month, last year.

Often the denial took the form of talking about an unrelated topic. The players would say a word or two in response to the diagnosis, there would be silence for a moment or two, and then the pair would begin to talk about other things. When I remonstrated mildly that they were not staying with the exercise, they protested that they had said all there was to say, and there was nothing more to role-play.

In contrast, a group of nursing students apparently found it difficult to "misunderstand" what the doctor was saying. More often they flatly rejected the diagnosis. Many then explained that they did not feel they would ever use denial after the initial response to shock. After the initial, "No! It couldn't be true!" they would quickly accept the reality of the diagnosis. They generally attributed this behavior to their professional education.

2. Responding to denial

To recognize the patient's denial, and to be able to duplicate denial behavior in an educational setting is only the beginning of skill in dealing with denial. A question often asked by health personnel is, what do you say when someone is engaged in denial? And, when you *do* decide on what to say, are you sure you are communicating what the patient needs to hear?

The following exercise may provide some answers. In the *Patient* column are statements of denial made by patients. The *Nurse* column contains possible responses. Pick the response that you believe would be most helpful to the patient and note why you chose it. If you decide that none of the choices are appropriate, note your reasons.

When everyone has finished all the items, get together and share the reasons for your choices. Afterwards, you might like to read some of my own observations on each of the items.

Patient says/does	*Nurse says/does*
1. "I can't believe it! It's not possible!"	A. "I'm sorry, but it's true. There's no doubt about it. As the doctor said, you have cancer." B. "Maybe you're right. Mistakes do happen." C. "Take your medication for now. It will make you feel better."
2. "This can't be happening to me."	A. "Everyone feels that way at first." B. Silence. After a while, *sit down* and say, "Do you have any questions you would like to ask me?"
3. "All kinds of mistakes are made here. Just yesterday, someone came in to get a sputum sample from me—and it turned out they were in the wrong room."	A. "Let's not be childish. We don't make mistakes about anything so serious." B. Silence. C. "Well, this is a big hospital. It's always possible."
4. "Those aren't my X-rays. I was just down there; they couldn't have developed them so quickly."	A. "X-rays can be developed in 10 minutes." B. "The doctor took other tests, too. He doesn't rely on X-rays alone." C. "X-rays need to be interpreted. They're not all that perfectly clear."
5. "I think the best thing to do is leave here and go to another doctor. I'm not satisfied with the explanation you are giving me."	A. "Four doctors examined you and the results of your tests. They can't all be wrong." B. "Why don't you wait and see how the medication makes you feel?" C. "Take your medicine and you'll be fine."

Patient says/does	*Nurse says/does*
6. This is the patient's third hospitalization—and third hospital. At each hospital she has left after the diagnosis, refusing treatment.	A. "You can't keep on wasting everyone's time this way. The doctors want to save your life, but you won't let them." B. Tell everyone about this patient—tell them not to exert themselves because she'll probaby leave before they can do anything for her. C. "Let us try to help you; at least to make you feel a little better."
7. "You're always reading about patients who outlive the doctors who told them they were dying. Just last week I read about a man of 98 who was told 50 years ago that he had only six months to live."	A. "I wouldn't want to live that long." B. "That's one case in a million. That's why it gets into the papers." C. "Things like that have happened occasionally."
8. "What's really got me flat on my back is this dizziness. As soon as they clear that up, I'll be fine."	A. "The dizziness is a minor thing. You're a very sick man, and you've got to accept that." B. "I'm sure you will." C. "Dizziness is certainly a disturbing symptom. The medication should help clear it up."
9. A patient who has been so hopeful and optimistic in discussing his future with you, has been talking to another nurse about his fear of dying.	A. "It would be better for you not to talk to Mr. Johns if he depresses you." B. "It's good to see you smiling and in good spirits. Don't ever get discouraged." C. "Are you so cheerful with me because you think that I don't care how you really feel?"
10. "Move that dressing table away from the foot of the bed. I don't have to keep looking at myself all the time."	A. "It's been there since you were admitted. What's so urgent about getting it moved now?" B. Move the table without comment. C. "Don't you want to see to fix yourself up for visitors?"
11. "Some day, I'll take my wife on that trip to Italy we've always talked about. We've planned and planned for it, but something has always interfered." *Later,* "Why should I undergo surgery again?	A. "You're contradicting yourself. One minute you're making plans to go to Italy and the next you're saying it's no use." B. "The surgery will help control the pain; you'll be more comfortable."

Patient says/does	*Nurse says/does*
It's no use. Just let me die in peace."	C. "You want to get to Italy, don't you? Then, you must follow doctor's orders."
12. "It's hard to die when your life hasn't even really begun. There was so much I still wanted to do. "This isn't the first time I've had to face a tough fight. I'll win through this like I did before."	A. "Of course you will. You're very brave." B. Bite lips; feel and look very uncomfortable. C. "I know how you must feel."
13. "I don't mind dying. I know my husband and child are waiting for me, and we'll be together again."	A. "That's right. You'll be happy again." B. "Do you really believe in that sort of thing?" C. Silence.
14. Patient turns away, refusing to respond to overtures.	A. Leave the patient to himself because he is not very pleasant or cooperative. B. Come back again and again, each time saying only, "I'm available when you want me." C. "Now you must talk about this. It's not good for you to keep it bottled up inside."
15. "I couldn't be as sick as they say. Once I get back to my own home, I'll be fine."	A. "How can you say that, when you know you can eat few things that don't make you deathly ill?" B. "I'm glad you're feeling better today. Keeping on your diet controls the nausea." C. "Of course you will!"

Discussion of the Exercise

1. A. Insisting immediately that "There is no doubt . . ." in the face of the patient's obvious need for denial is not helpful. Trying to force someone to believe something is usually not a very productive strategy for learning. Especially when the information to be learned has an enormous affective component, the chances are that the person being forced will: (1) close himself off to further communication by withdrawing; (2) take a firm stand in rejecting the validity of the information, bringing to bear all kinds of experiences and data to bolster his position;

(3) or respond with such great anxiety and perturbation that it is obvious that the information will not be used to help himself.

1. B. Going along with the patient's denial and even reinforcing it by offering additional data is so easy to do that it suggests the nurse may be responding to her own needs rather than to the patient's. If the nurse's objective is to give the patient time to absorb and accept the fact of his dying, then it is useless to assure him that his denial is entirely appropriate. Agreement will make dying much more difficult for him to accept. Encouraging the patient's denial may be motivated by *one's own* inability to accept the fact of dying.

1. C. Neither reinforcing nor rejecting the patient's denial implies an acceptance—not of the denial, perhaps, but of his need for it. Offering the medication indicates that the nurse accepts the person, too, regardless of what he happens to be saying at the moment. The nurse is also able to focus on something real; the medicine *will* make the patient feel better. Although the total reality is too much for the patient to accept now, he is exposed to at least part of the reality—a hopeful part.

2. A. In our society, where information is so highly valued, it is always tempting to tell what we know to people who do *not* know. Parents are forever trying to prevent their children from making the same mistakes the parent made, and they feel that the way to do this is to tell the children what parents learned long ago. Teachers are probably the worst offenders. They think that teaching means telling children the information the teachers have been able to gather in their lifetimes. Given this kind of orientation, it is no surprise that so many of us fall into this pattern: telling what we know every chance we get.

When the nurse tells the patient, "Everyone feels that way at first," he or she is trying to force the patient to give up denial. But the nurse does this in a particular way: recalling what he or she has learned from Dr. Kübler-Ross about the stages of dying, the nurse is telling the patient, in effect, "You are just going through a stage." The nurse implies that the patient's feelings are not that important: he is just going through a phase that every dying patient goes through.

2. B. Silence neither reinforces denial nor interferes with the patient's need to deny. However, silence may be misinterpreted. For example, when the patient protests that this cannot be happening to him, the nurse may choose to say nothing and leave the bedside. Her behavior in this case may be easily interpreted as disapproval, or avoidance of discomfort. If silence is to be effective, it must accompany eye contact between patient and nurse and may even involve physical contact: holding the patient's hand or rubbing his arm.

After a mutual silence, the nurse may encourage the patient to begin to accept his illness. The nurse may give him a chance to ask questions, and, by *sitting down,* make it clear that he is prepared to answer the questions; this will help reassure the patient that he will not be left alone to cope with his feelings of shock and fear.

3. A. Here, not only is the nurse trying to force the patient to give up his denial, but he is acting in a rather pejorative way, denigrating him, making it clear that his behavior is disapproved of. Thus, the punishment is added to the burden the patient already bears. Actually, the response sounds rather defensive, as if the attack on the hospital were a personal attack on the nurse. Here the nurse's need apparently takes precedence over the patient's need.

3. B. This is accepting behavior, bearing in mind the warning in 2. B.

3. C. This response smacks of catering to one's own need for denial, or at least a need to avoid dealing with the reality of dying.

4. A. This information forces the patient to face reality. Telling the patient how long it takes to develop an X-ray is irrelevant.

4. B. The nurse adopts a "no-nonsense" approach, insisting quite abruptly that the patient be realistic. The patient is not given time to face the truth.

4. C. This response seems to give the patient a further opportunity to avoid reality for a longer time. Again, although the nurse might maintain that he is saying this out of sympathy for the patient's anguish, he may actually be responding out of his own need to avoid dealing openly with the patient's dying.

5. A. This response attempts to force the patient into a quick acceptance.

5. B. Offering reality in a hopeful way is both honest and helpful. Medication may help, even if it does not cure. There is no encouragement of flight from the facts, nor is there an attempt to back the patient into a corner and force-feed him the whole truth.

5. C. Promising cure to a terminally ill patient is fostering and supporting denial.

6. A. This is a curious response to the patient's denial behavior, having a number of different effects. It is moralizing in a punitive way, with the possibility that it will make the patient feel guilty (". . . wasting everyone's time . . ."). It adds to the guilt by putting the blame for dying on the patient (". . . you won't let them. . ."). It tries to force the patient to give up his denial behavior, yet also encourages him to maintain his denial by making a strong implication that if he does what the doctors say he will not die.

6. B. Here the nurse is responding to the patient's denial with anger. He is using his knowledge of the patient's behavior in the past to encourage the health personnel to expect difficulty from the patient. This can be a very effective way to deter them from trying out new strategies for

reaching the patient—strategies that might help him finally to face his illness realistically. Surely there is no point in trying to help someone who will leave before you can succeed with him!

6. C. This answer provides a little reality with some hope: a step in the direction of peace.

7. A. This is a glib remark, a weak attempt at humor, almost sarcastic in tone. Responding this way to a patient's serious clutching at unrealistic optimism can only make him angry. It can also retard the development of trust between nurse and patient: not many people expect to have a trusting relationship with someone who makes them the butt of humor.

7. B. The patient's hope here is, of course, unrealistic, and the example she gives merely bolsters his denial. However, to destroy that hope so abruptly, is to precipitate the kind of behavior that forcing does.

7. C. On the other hand, mildly admitting that things like that happen occasionally—as they do—demonstrates acceptance of the patient's need for denial, points out the rarity of the occurrence (this is reality), and avoids giving additional strength to the denial.

8. A. At the moment, the patient is obviously made very uncomfortable by the dizziness. To tell him at this time that it is not important is really not helpful. He would seem to have enough to cope with at the moment without immediately facing the fact that he is dying.

8. B. Agreeing with the patient completely encourages him to extend the time of denying, and incidentally, gets the nurse off the hook.

8. C. Certainly, the nurse here responds to one of the patient's immediate needs—reassurance that the disturbing symptom can be alleviated. The nurse is careful not to agree with the patient's denial by accepting that he will be fine when the dizziness goes away. However, perhaps there *is* an element of avoidance on the part of the nurse: might the patient easily be misled into believing that the nurse agrees with him? Should the nurse be a little clearer about exactly what the medicine will and will not do?

9. A. The nurse assumes that expressing his feelings depresses the patient. It is very likely that *she* is the one who would feel depressed if she talked with the patient openly about his dying. She is probably determinedly cheerful in his presence, making it quite clear that she does not want him to talk about anything "depressing." The patient has read the message and is going along with it; he saves his honesty for the person who is ready to accept it and respond in kind—Mr. Johns.

9. B. The nurse in this example doesn't dare to recognize that the patient *is* talking openly with someone else. This kind of behavior is what makes denial so difficult to deal with; not only must we recognize and cope productively with the patient's denial, but we must also recognize and deal with our own need to avoid facing death.

You may have noticed that I use the word *denial* when talking about the patient, and generally use *avoidance* when referring to the behavior of health personnel. This is because I do think there is a difference in the two responses. The patient's denial indicates—even if only temporarily and sporadically—that the patient really *believes* that he is not dying. On the other hand, the nurse generally believes no such thing when she purposefully avoids the subject of death. Taking into consideration all the possible questions about "What does *believing* mean?" and "Can a person believe on one level of awareness and not on another?" I would still say that there is a significant difference between the patient's and the nurse's awareness.

9. C. If the nurse becomes aware of the message she has been sending the patient by her behavior, she can tell him that she is ready to relate to him honestly. Notice there is no accusation here: why do you talk to him, but not to me? The statement is merely an opening to permit the nurse to demonstrate a different behavior if the patient will trust her.

10. A. This type of logic has the effect of forcing the patient to recognize that he is denying the fact of his dying. (It may be that she is reluctant to look at herself in the mirror because in it she sees the unmistakable signs of her illness. Not looking may, for a while, keep awareness at a distance.) It is obvious that the nurse neither appreciates nor accepts the patient's denial.

10. B. By moving the table the nurse accepts the patient's denial. The nurse realizes the patient's appearance is deteriorating; if the patient is ready to do so, he may read this message too, and begin to face the implications.

10. C. The patient does not look the way she did when she was healthy. To suggest that she will is not realistic.

11. A. Pointing out contradictions is an attempt to force the patient to give up his denial behavior. A person cannot think about death all the time. Often, he may think about other things so completely that for a moment he feels that he is not dying after all. He has a right to this respite.

11. B. Being specific about the probable effects of surgery does not mislead the patient into believing that he will be well. The response offers the patient a reality without pain, but no more.

11. C. This response reinforces the patient's denial by providing false hope. It also takes unfair advantage of the patient's denial to force him to accept a recommendation for surgery. And, incidentally, it helps the nurse avoid dealing with the inevitability of death.

12. A. This comment fosters denial and avoids openness.

12. B. The nurse seems to have been caught unaware, unable to accept the denial, and having no way to respond without causing even greater

discomfort. He probably has not had enough experience in communicating with dying people to develop effective avoidance behavior, so he stays and becomes more and more uncomfortable.

12. C. "I know how you must feel," is a response to the first part of the patient's statement. The nurse so obviously ignores the second part that the patient is practically forced to realize that the nurse disagrees with his belief that he will not die.

13. A. Believing that life continues after death is a kind of denial of death—a kind that might be shared by the nurse and patient in this instance. However, the expression of such a belief does not necessarily mean the patient is spared the fear and anger and other emotions associated with the awareness of dying. The responsibility of the medical practitioner in continuing effective interaction is not fulfilled just because the patient and nurse agree on the existence of life after death.

13. B. The nurse questions life after death and the patient's belief.

13. C. Perhaps the most effective response in this situation is to simply listen to the patient's beliefs and feelings. There will be other opportunities for helping the patient deal productively with his illness.

14. A. Is the nurse relieved not to have to confront the fact of death with the patient? She is certainly quick to react to symptoms (unpleasantness, uncooperativeness) and ignore the problem (shock, denial).

14 B. This is accepting. The patient needs to know that the people around him will not abandon him. He needs to be constantly reassured that they are ready to respond to him *when he needs them*. It is the *patient* who must set the pace for the process called dying.

14. C. This response attempts to force the patient.

15. A. Obviously, this is a no-nonsense, forcing approach to make the patient aware of his dying.

15. B. This is the reality reference: You feel better today; keeping on the diet helps; but (implied) what we're talking about is now, and the symptom; we cannot talk about going home or being well. If the patient is ready to hear this message, it is there for him.

15. C. This statement encourages denial and avoidance.

chapter four

———◄◄◆►►———

Anger

Identifying the stage

Kübler-Ross's next stage in the dying process is anger. Of course, dying people do not necessarily go in an orderly fashion from one predetermined stage to another, clearly presenting at each stage specific behaviors that were never seen in earlier stages and will never again be seen once the current stage has run its course. Fear may be an undercurrent emotion from the day of the first symptom to the day of the last breath, and denial may alternate with completely open awareness. A patient may begin to bargain with the fates immediately after the initial shock of knowledge is over; anger may flare up again and again, triggered each time by a different individual or occurrence.

Unlike denial behavior, anger is not socially approved. In our culture, the angry child is often punished for impertinence. The angry adult is often labeled "immature." For some people, to be angry in the face of death almost has connotations of blasphemy, so at odds is this emotion with the denial and sentimentality with which we surround our communication about death.

Sometimes, it may be the husband or wife of the patient who provokes resentment and anger, fear and guilt; sometimes it is the mother or the child. Part of the patient's anger may be attributed to the pressure to pretend during visits that she is not dying. She tries to "protect" her family and they try to "protect" her from the knowledge that both of them have. The strain of the pretense alone is enough to create great tension and cause sighs of relief when visiting hours are over.

The patient may feel resentment that she must keep quiet about something very important that is happening to her. Most likely, she needs an opportunity to sort out her conflicting feelings and needs and come to a decision that will make interaction with her family more comfortable. The patient may find it easier to do this sorting out with a nurse than with a person with whom she is more emotionally involved.

Thus, the nurse who says to her, "How happy you must be to have a family who rallies around you when you need them!" may merely force her to keep quiet about how *un*happy that "rallying-around" is making her. Conversely, the nurse who says, "You seem to be uncomfortable when your mother comes to visit," and then just waits, may encourage the patient to feel that she can freely express her feelings without fear of censure. Of course, the nurse must be careful to make an objective observation and not an evaluation.

Some of the fear when facing loved ones may be attributed to the feeling that facing a loved one is like facing the reality of imminent loss. The look in his eyes, the pain that creases his brow, his apparent discomfort and sadness, his eagerness to placate all expressions of the patient's anger and to provide for every presumed physical need all remind the patient that she will not long have this loved one.

The patient may sometimes need to say—without feeling guilty—"I need to be alone for a while, to come to terms with what is happening to me. I can't cope with myself and with you too, right now." The nurse who says, "Is there something you'd like me to tell your family?" provides an opportunity for the patient to ask the nurse to intercede and ask the family not to visit so often for a while.

It is true that the patient may not take advantage of the opportunity, except to pour out her feelings of fear and anxiety and anger against her family. But her pouring-out may make it easier to live through another visit, knowing that it is not necessary to maintain the pretense with everyone, and that there will be time and help for coping when the visit is over.

Values and anger

Without being aware of what we are doing, we can make it clear that we hold certain values and assume that others hold those values too. In this way, we may imply to others that if they do not feel the way we do we will disapprove of them and of their behavior.

Suppose that a nurse has a 30-year-old woman patient whose obviously devoted husband visits her every morning, and twice on the day he is off from work. Before each daily visit, the nurse tells the patient, "Your husband will be here soon. Let me help you freshen up for him. You want to look your best, don't you?" Perhaps she might also say, "He's so devoted to you. You're lucky to have a husband like that."

A group of nurses were asked what the nurse in this instance wished to communicate to her patient. Here are their answers:

- that she approved of the patient's husband
- that a wife should always present a pleasant appearance to her husband
- that wives need to do a little pretending to keep their husbands interested
- that a wife shouldn't neglect her appearance despite how she feels
- that a woman is lucky to have an attentive husband
- that a woman shouldn't feel anything but appreciation for such a husband

It does seem that the nurse is trying to be helpful and to assure her patient that people care about her. However, the nurse is also making it very clear that the patient should appreciate so exemplary a husband and look forward eagerly to his visits.

But what if this woman, in fact, does *not* look forward to seeing her husband? What if she thinks about him with anger, and wishes only that he leave her alone? These feelings overwhelm and frighten her. She almost hates the man with whom she has always had a good relationship, and though she resents him now, she is also afraid of being abandoned in her illness. How can she discuss her feelings with a nurse who obviously appreciates her husband and sees nothing in his behavior to justify the wife's rejection? Wouldn't that nurse think her patient was unreasonable —and perhaps make her patient feel guilty?

An Exercise in Non-Judgmental Responses

Try to think of some of the things you, as a nurse, could say to this patient that: 1) would not reveal your own values or feelings about the husband and his relationship with his wife, 2) would clearly communicate your desire to help the patient physically, and 3) would communicate that you are ready to listen to whatever the patient wants to say without making any kind of a judgment. Perhaps you might check out your probable responses with the rest of your class. You may find that when you think you are being non-judgmental, other people are detecting your values and feelings.

For example, when you say, "Wouldn't you like me to help you get out of that hospital gown and put on your pretty nightgown?" you may be offering help, but you are also saying, "I think it's only natural that you should want to look attractive for your husband." If the patient feels differently, you may be adding to her fears that she is "unnatural" and to her feelings of guilt.

Saying, "You seem to be feeling a little down today. Don't worry, that husband of yours will cheer you up. He's really something, isn't he? He makes everyone on the floor feel good with his joking and kidding," doesn't help a patient who can only wish that her husband would not be so cheerful and amiable, but would sit quietly and hold her hand. But how can she say this to someone who thinks her husband's behavior is just right? The nurse might come to dislike her, think her ungrateful, maybe even see her as an uncooperative patient.

Here are some of the suggestions made by nurses that seem to fulfill the criterion of offering aid without making a judgment:

> "Things are a little quiet now. Is there some way I can be of help to you?"

> "Before the visitors descend on us, is there anything you need from me?"

> "It's good to have a few minutes relief from running. Would you like to talk a little while?"

One person felt that the nurse should be more directive, giving the patient a clue that her feelings would be empathically received. She would have said to the patient, "My husband is a great guy, but there are times when I'd like to kick him, he makes me so mad!" Of course, the effectiveness of this approach depends on the accuracy with which the nurse has interpreted the patient's feelings. The person who made the suggestion felt that by revealing something personal about herself without fear of rejection or condemnation she might encourage the patient to do the same. She also hastened to say that her remark would have to be honest, not merely contrived. And she also stressed the importance of restraining herself from discussing details of her own problem instead of being quiet and letting the patient do the talking.

Practicing anger

Suppose that a week ago Mrs. Smith, a woman of thirty-five, discovered that she was terminally ill. Since then she has been alternately denying her imminent death and lashing out in anger at everyone around her. Miss Jones, a student nurse, has been assigned to her. It is a beautiful spring day and Miss Jones has enjoyed her short walk to work and is ready to do a good job. She comes up to Mrs. Smith's bed and smiles brightly. "Good morning, Mrs. Smith. I'm Ellie Jones. I'll be taking care of you today. How are you feeling?"

"Oh, fine. Just fine," answers Mrs. Smith, gritting her teeth. "Since you'll be *taking care* of me today, would you mind pulling that window shade down? Why can't I get you people to understand?! I want the shade *down!*"

What happens now?

If you think you have some idea of what Mrs. Smith is feeling, you play the role of Mrs. Smith. Someone else will be Miss Jones. Now pick up the action at the point where the story stops and play it out for a few minutes. While you are doing this, the rest of the class observes and takes notes.

In their enactment, how does Miss Jones respond to Mrs. Smith's anger? Are her feelings obviously hurt? Does she say or do anything to reveal her own feelings? Does Miss Jones try to correct the things that are making Mrs. Smith angry? How successful is she in satisfying Mrs. Smith?

Play and re-play the parts with different people and after each role-play discuss what you have observed. You might keep in mind, as you interact in the role-playing, what the researchers have observed about the anger of dying patients: "the issue is often totally irrelevant." "staff or family reacts personally . . . only feeding into the patient's hostile behavior." (Kübler-Ross, *On Death and Dying*, p. 52). You might decide that you feel too uncomfortable responding in a particular way, and that you could *never* do so, no matter what *anybody* said. Here is a good opportunity for you to "try on" the kind of behavior you are unaccustomed to. Here, in the safety of the classroom, you can risk behaving in a way that is new for you. You may find it more comfortable than you expect, and you may get responses that are so satisfying that you will be willing to try the new behavior again.

Discussion

You may find that, no matter how hard Miss Jones tries to fulfill the patient's requests, she remains angry. As a matter of fact, her anger may increase until it includes everyone who has contact with her.

Miss Jones may finally throw up her hands in disgust and leave Mrs.

Smith alone. She won't be in a hurry to answer when her light goes on again!

Or Miss Jones may say, "Really, Mrs. Smith, you're being unreasonable! Everyone is doing their best to make you comfortable, and you appreciate nothing! If you're not careful, people will begin avoiding you. Do you want to be left completely alone, with nobody coming to see you at all?"

Perhaps Miss Jones, in this case, is one of those motherly yet firm people who will take no nonsense from patients. She may make it clear to Mrs. Smith that she was behaving childishly and must stop such behavior at once.

How does Mrs. Smith feel about these different responses to her anger? Is she sorry she's being difficult? Does her anger increase so that she has room for no other emotion—like fear, for example? Is it possible that the more she is threatened with isolation, the more frightened she becomes, and the more she goads herself to anger?

Does she continue her condemnation of the staff, the physical surroundings, and even her own family? Does she burst into tears? Does she turn her face to the wall? Does she threaten to leave the hospital?

Or Miss Jones may quietly draw the blind, help make Mrs. Smith as comfortable as she can, physically, and then reassure her by saying, "Whenever you want me, I'll be available."

How would these different responses make Mrs. Smith feel? Would any of them allay her anger? Her fear?

Ultimately, you may conclude there is no way of being sure that a particular behavior is always appropriate in a particular situation. Of course, no two people respond the same way; you will have to judge your own responses to see if they help or hurt an angry patient.

Identifying differential responses to anger

Below are twenty things that patients may say or do which express their anger. Under each expression of anger are various responses a nurse might make to an angry patient. In the columns at the right, each response is checked to indicate that the nurse (a) accepts the patient's anger, (b) encourages the patient to express his anger, (c) expresses the nurse's anger, or (d) reveals the nurse's fear.

Cover the columns with a sheet of paper and decide in which column you would classify each of the responses by the nurse. Later, your answers may be compared to those in the book. The footnote symbols next to certain check marks indicate there are comments on that particular item.

	a) Acceptance	b) Encouragement	c) Anger	d) Fear
PATIENT: "I've asked you a hundred times not to put the cover over my feet!" (Kicks cover off.) "Just go away, will you!"				
NURSE: (Turns abruptly and leaves the room.)			√	√ [1]
(Tucks the covers in tightly around the bed.)			√	
"I'm sorry. I don't know where my head is!"	√			
"I hate people doing things to me too. I don't blame you for sounding off!"		√		
PATIENT: "Would you mind talking *to* me, instead of about me? I'm not dead yet, you know!"				
NURSE: "Of course you're not! Don't talk that way!"				√ [2]
"These are professional matters that patients don't understand."				√ [2]
(Ignores the patient and continues talking.)				
"Sorry, we didn't mean to do that." (Changes the subject to casual conversation and includes the patient.)				√ [3]
"Sorry, we were talking about a change in your medication. You've been complaining about increasing pain, and we want to make sure you are reasonably comfortable all the time."	√			
PATIENT: "I felt a lot better before I got mixed up with all of you. What are you doing—using me for a guinea pig?"				
NURSE: "How can you suggest such a thing! Here we are, doing all we can to help you, and you accuse us of unethical behavior!"				√ [4]
"Now, you *know* you're very sick, and *that's* why you feel bad. You can't say that we're making you sick!"				√ [4]
PATIENT: "How long must I wait before someone answers the bell? I hear you all sitting out there having a fine time! Why don't you do your job?"				

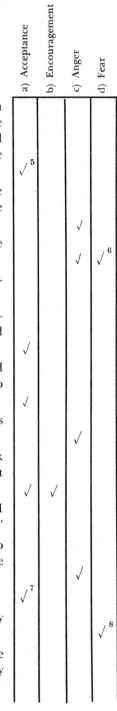

	a) Acceptance	b) Encouragement	c) Anger	d) Fear

NURSE: "Would it help if I promised to look in on you every time I have a free minute? That will be every half-hour or so; if your ring isn't answered immediately by someone else, you can feel sure that I'll come in a few minutes." — √ 5

"You'll just have to wait your turn like everyone else. You're not the only sick person on the floor!" — √ (Anger)

(She comes in less and less often—ignoring the ring as much as possible.) — √ (Anger) √ 6 (Fear)

PATIENT: "I am *Mrs. Smith* to you. And don't you forget it!"

NURSE: "I'm sorry. I feel more comfortable when people are less formal. I just assumed you would feel that way too." — √ (Acceptance)

"You're right: we get into the habit around here of using patients' first names. We ought to ask permission first." — √ (Acceptance)

"We call all patients by their first names. It's more convenient." — √ (Anger)

"You're right to get angry. I hope you'll speak out about things that bug you around here. It will help us help you." — √ (Acceptance) √ (Encouragement)

PATIENT: "Get out of here! I didn't send for you—I have enough people pawing over me already!"

NURSE: "You really are ungrateful! You'll fix it so no one will want to come in here and try to make you comfortable!" — √ (Anger)

"I'll be here when you want me." — √ 7 (Acceptance)

"If you don't let us help you, you'll have only yourself to blame for not getting well!" — √ 8 (Fear)

PATIENT: "The doctors here don't know what they're doing! I can't get a straight answer out of any of them!"

	a) Acceptance	b) Encouragement	c) Anger	d) Fear
NURSE: "Everyone is doing his best to help you. You must stay calm and do as you're told."				√9
"Tell me what you want to know, and maybe I can get answers for you."	√10	√10		
(Sits down and makes it clear that she is ready to listen.)	√	√		
"The doctors here are the best in the country! If you had to pay one-half of the cost of the care you're getting, you'd realize how good they are!"			√	
PATIENT: "The level of efficiency here is zero! If I ran my business the way they run this hospital, I'd have been bankrupt years ago!"				
NURSE: "You don't have to deal with sick people in your business! Sick people are not always reasonable!"			√	
(Bursts into tears.)				√11
(Nods sympathetically and listens.)			√	
PATIENT: "I told you I didn't want any visitors! Can't you leave me in peace!"				
NURSE: "Call me when you want me—any time."	√			
"All right! If you want to be alone, we'll leave you alone!"			√	
"I'll suggest that people call you before they come, so you can tell them if you feel like having visitors."	√	√		
"I notice there are some visitors you don't object to. Can you tell me what makes them more comfortable to have around?"		√12		
PATIENT: "Jones will really be happy now! The S.O.B. has been after my job for years!"				
NURSE: "Oh, I can't believe that people are as mean as you make them out to be."				√13
"This man Jones—what is he like?"	√	√14		

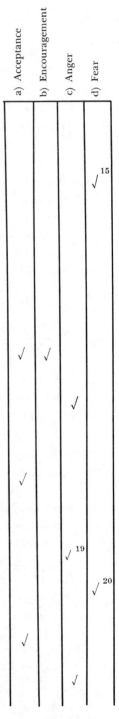

	a) Acceptance	b) Encouragement	c) Anger	d) Fear

PATIENT: "Will you keep this old man (Mr. Smith in the next bed) quiet! I don't want to hear about his grandchildren!"

NURSE: "I'll put the curtains around your bed so you won't have to talk to him." $\checkmark$ [15]

"Now, he isn't hurting you. Just behave yourself and try to get along.[16]

"Did you know that Mr. Smith lives in your neighborhood? He was telling me about the trash collection problem you mentioned yesterday." [17]

PATIENT: I'm not ready for a bath now! I'll bathe when *I'm* ready!"

NURSE: "I can understand your anger. I'd hate to have people controlling everything I do." $\checkmark$ $\checkmark$

"I'm sorry, but you're not my only patient! You'll just have to follow the schedule like everyone else." $\checkmark$

"Let me leave the basin here with hot water in it. By the time you're ready, it will be cool enough for you to use. Just ring if you need some help." [18] $\checkmark$

PATIENT: (Shoves the nurse's hand away when she attempts to administer medication.)

NURSE: "You do that again and I'll tie you down if I have to!" $\checkmark$ [19]

(Insists that the charge nurse or the physician administer medication for this patient.) $\checkmark$ [20]

"The medicine will ease your pain and make you more comfortable. Please let us help you as much as we can." $\checkmark$

"When you hurt badly enough, you can ask *me* for medication!" $\checkmark$

	a) Acceptance	b) Encouragement	c) Anger	d) Fear
"You have no right to interfere this way with the treatment! You have a responsibility to your family and to the people who are trying to help you.				√ [21]
PATIENT: (Throws the water pitcher on the floor.)				
NURSE: "I ought to make you mop it up! You're acting like a baby!"			√	
"The pitcher isn't a bad thing to throw when you get mad. It's unbreakable."	√			
"If you feel like getting it off your chest, I have some time to listen."		√		
"You're inconsiderate—you make more work for all of us because you have no self-control."			√	
PATIENT: (Turns impatiently to the wall when the nurse speaks to him.)			√ [22]	√ [22]
NURSE: (Doesn't attempt to speak to him again; does her work efficiently and leaves.)				
"Please remember that I'm available to talk whenever you feel like it."	√			
(Make a point of coming in regularly and sitting down for a few minutes, making it clear each time that she has time to talk—and listen—for a little while. Do this again and again, until you hit on a time when the patient is ready to talk.)	√	√		
PATIENT: (Stares at the nurse belligerently when she asks a question.)				
NURSE: "You needn't be so unpleasant about it; I'm only trying to help you."			√	
(Delays answering the patient's calls.)			√	
"You look so angry." (Stated calmly.)		√		
Silence.				√ [23]

	a) Acceptance	b) Encouragement	c) Anger	d) Fear
PATIENT: (Pulls abruptly away when the nurse touches her.)				
NURSE: (Feels hurt and avoids touching the patient in the future.)			√	
"I was just trying to let you know that I'm here whenever you want me."		√		
"There are times when I hate having people touch me. When you're a patient, you probably get more of it than you want."	√	√		
PATIENT: (Deliberately tears the pages of a book to shreds.)				
NURSE: "What a destructive, childish thing to do!"			√	
"You're very angry, aren't you."	√	√		
(Ignores the behavior.)				√
PATIENT: (Refuses to follow medical orders that may prolong his life.)				
NURSES "You have no right to do as you please. You have a responsibility to the people who are trying to help you and to your family."				√ 21
"You will make yourself feel worse by not following your diet."	√ 24			
"I know you're angry and frustrated about this. Anyone would be."		√		
PATIENT: (Begins to put on his clothes and refuses to respond when the nurse protests.)				
NURSE: "You walk out of here and you'll be committing suicide!"			√	√
"Don't be childish; act your age."			√	
"I know you're angry and hurt. Sit down and talk a while before you rush out."	√	√		

Discussion

1. The nurse who is disturbed at the prospect of this patient's imminent death may be afraid to respond to his anger. Her response may let loose a flood of feelings about dying that the nurse would rather avoid.
2. Usually the attempts to maintain a wall of noncommunication between patient and health-care personnel are based on fear. The nurse or physician who maintains that he keeps information from the patient because the patient cannot understand the technicalities of the disease or the treatment is afraid of being seen as a fallible human being, afraid of committing himself to a human relationship with all that this implies in the way of accepting and expressing feelings, afraid of having himself open to the patient's questions. In more superficial terms, it is downright rude to talk about a person as if he were not there.

   This kind of behavior is observable not only among medical personnel vis-à-vis patient; teachers and parents demonstrate similar behavior in their dealings with children, and, in a way, employers do this to employees. Such behavior has a dehumanizing effect, denying the feelings of the person thus used. Those who resist such dehumanization may quite understandably do so with anger and resentment.
3. The medical personnel fear upsetting the dying patient by persisting in a behavior that annoys him. At the same time they are reluctant to discuss his condition with him—perhaps for fear of telling him too much. The end result is an obviously patronizing compromise— they include him only in talk about trivialities.
4. The nurse responds by defending herself and the rest of the staff against what she feels is an unfair attack. The mistake she makes is believing that this is the real issue involved. It is much more likely that the patient's attack is actually a displacement of anger and frustration about dying. Dealing with the *apparent* object of attack does not help the patient.
5. Sometimes anger is a function of the panic a patient feels when he believes that no one will respond quickly enough should he need someone desperately. Acceptance of his anger and a plan for reassuring him may help.
6. This behavior seems to be retaliation for the patient's insult. However, this kind of response to a dying patient is often a function of fear: the nurse realizes the patient is struggling with the fact of his dying and is fearful of having to confront this fact sooner or later.

If there is sustained interaction between patient and nurse, it may become increasingly difficult to maintain the fiction that the patient will return to health. The nurse, by avoiding such interaction, also avoids the possibility of being asked a direct question about dying or having to respond to an explicit statement about dying.

7. The patient is angry at the moment, furious at the overwhelming knowledge that he is dying. However, he is also frightened, and he needs to know that when some of his anger has subsided and he needs someone to listen and to care, that someone will be available.

8. The nurse is well aware that the patient will not recover. Here he seems to be trying to allay his own anxiety about failing to maintain health and life by shifting the "blame" to the patient.

9. The nurse avoids responding to the need of the patient, who is demanding more open and honest communication. This may be another instance of a "conspiracy" to keep the fact of his dying from the patient. In this case, the stated objective is probably to keep the patient hopeful and cheerful; the real objective is probably to save the medical personnel from the discomfort of having to discuss the patient's dying with him. Perhaps, the doctors and nurses are avoiding the reality of death because of their own anxieties, thereby increasing the anxiety and frustration of the patient!

10. It is not easy for the nurse to take the initiative in being honest with the patient when doctors and, perhaps, family members want to maintain silence. However, in recognizing the problem the others are having, the nurse is strategically situated to feed back to them factual information about the patient's behavior and so to encourage them to re-examine their decision. For example, she can make it clear that the patient knows more about his illness than he has been told, and that their silence is making him suffer from anxiety and frustration. In any case, she can offer to be the one to talk with him if none of the others are able to do so.

11. It is possible that if this were not a dying patient, the nurse would respond with anger, telling him in no uncertain terms that *he* was the kind of patient who interfered with hospital efficiency. However, torn between her anger with an unpleasant patient and her fear of being honest with a dying person, her response is one of frustration and helplessness—tears.

12. Perhaps the patient finds he can talk more honestly about his illness and dying with only certain people. If the nurse finds this is true, perhaps she can emulate the behavior of those people and become another person who can be of help to the patient.

13. Most likely, her fear of death and dying compels the nurse to respond in this unrealistic and unhelpful manner. Perhaps many people are

reluctant to believe that, in the face of the awful reality of death, anyone would actually be pleased. (In the face of the awful reality of *our own* death, how distasteful to contemplate that some people may be pleased!)

14. This response encourages the patient to express his strong hostile feelings, without fear of condemnation. Whether or not the patient's anger against Jones is justified, a sympathetic, non-judgmental listener may give him some immediate relief and permit him—in his own time —to allow the anger to subside.

15. There seems to be a reluctance on the part of the nurse to confront the patient face to face. She overlooks the fact that the patient's anger —although apparently directed against the man in the next bed—is really a generalized anger that cannot be lessened by punishing the other man (isolating him behind the curtain) or by letting the patient isolate himself. The nurse feels more comfortable in avoiding the whole issue.

16. Some of these professional responses do not belong in any of the columns. It is difficult to classify a response like this one, perhaps, because it reveals no intensity of feeling, or any specific attempt to be helpful. If it reveals anything, it is that the nurse is just ignoring the other person's feelings and using her authority to silence him.

17. This response doesn't recognize the patient's anger. Rather, the nurse seems to ignore the patient's feeling, and tries to divert him by encouraging interaction with the other man. If the patient's anger is deep-seated, the attempt will prove futile. (Can *you* chit-chat with someone when you're furious?)

18. It is sometimes helpful in allaying anger to provide opportunity for the patient to maintain a measure of control over his own life wherever possible. It can be extremely disturbing for an active self-directed person to suddenly have his whole life ordered by others. He is often controlled more in the interest of some idea of hospital efficiency than because his illness demands it.

19. The reaction is an almost violent assertion of the traditional professional role (administering medication)—perhaps to avoid dealing with the fear of inevitable death.

20. It seems that the nurse is reluctant to come into any kind of direct confrontation with this patient. Can it be that she is torn between pity that he is dying, fear that he may say something about it (like "What's the use of all this medicine? I'm going to die anyhow!"), and guilt that medical science really cannot help him?

21. Such righteous indignation seems to be an attempt to shift the burden of guilt to the patient. The nurse knows very well that following orders will not prolong the patient's life, but she cannot confront

this fact. She feels helpless, guilty, and afraid, and here may be trying
to make the patient bear some of the guilt.

22. Perhaps the nurse is relieved at not having to speak to the patient.
Her relief may be based on fear that communication will inevitably
bring up the topic of death. Feeling guilty about this relief may
easily lead to anger—the kind of righteous anger that makes a person
say: "It's not *my* fault that you're isolated! You brought that on yourself by your behavior!"

23. Silence may ensue because of wariness in relating to a dying person.
For fear of disturbing the patient further, the nurse may keep interaction to a minimum.

24. The nurse accepts the patient's anger, but manages to hold before
his eyes a reality reference. That is, it is quite true that maintaining
his diet makes the patient feel better. This is not to reject him, or
his anger; only, perhaps, to start to encourage him to deal with his
anger in a more productive way.

chapter five

———◀◆▶———

Bargaining

Identifying the stage

Kübler-Ross states that dying people arrive at the bargaining stage in an attempt to postpone the inevitable (p. 83). If their lives can only be extended until they can do the one thing they have always wanted to do, or make amends for something they have regretted doing, or see again someone they have been separated from for a long time, then they promise they will give in to death. Sometimes the patients are able to do or to see what they have bargained for. There are times when the wish is so strong that it seems actually to prolong a life until it is fulfilled.

Too often, however, hospital personnel do not seem to take these wishes seriously, despite their importance to the patient. Sometimes the wishes are rather forcefully rejected by logical arguments to prove that the patient is not being reasonable.

There are no set answers for helping a patient when he is involved in bargaining for a little more life or a little less pain. But maybe we can, by reaching inside ourselves, find resources for appreciating the unfulfilled wishes and yearnings of others. Perhaps out of such appreciation will come the words and the behavior for helping people to die with acceptance.

An Exercise in Appreciation

Sit in a circle with your colleagues. Each person should have five to ten blank cards. Imagine you have been told that you do not have very long to live. What are the things that you would love to do before you die?

Write each wish on a separate card and put the cards into the middle of the circle. When everyone has finished, shuffle the cards so that the authors cannot be identified. Put the stack of cards face down in the center of the circle.

One person at a time may draw a card and read it aloud. The participants should spend about five minutes discussing why each wish is important to the person who wrote it. No one during the discussion should suggest that the wish is not important, or that it is less important than something else. The objective is to focus on the importance of this to the person who wrote it, and it may require some mental gymnastics to project yourselves into the mind and heart of someone to whom this particular thing was so important that he reached for it as one of his last wishes on earth.

The author of the card may participate in the discussion and offer insights that the others may not have. However, he need not identify himself as the writer unless he chooses to do so. It works best if—should he choose to identify himself—he leaves this until the discussion has gone on for some time, so that what he has to say can serve as a check on the perceptions and observations of the others.

Discussion

One group of students who participated in this exercise responded nervously to their present situation. They were studying for mid-semester examinations and felt the usual anxiety about passing, as well as anger against certain instructors who did not seem aware of the problems they were causing. One student wrote that if she *knew* she were dying, she would take the opportunity to tell a certain anatomy instructor what she thought of him. Another student wanted to eat her fill of marshmallow cookies before she died.

One woman remembered an injustice she thought she had committed against her mother years ago. She had never discussed it with anyone, nor had the opportunity to ask her mother's forgiveness before the latter's death. Now she felt that, if she herself were faced with imminent death, she would want enough time to come to some sense of peace over the incident.

One young man felt he could not let himself die until he had provided financial security for his wife and child. The nursing instructor in the group said she would want desperately to finish the book she was writing before she died. An older woman wanted to attend her son's graduation from college. A young woman wanted time—and help—in becoming friends with her older sister again.

An Exercise in Responding with Appreciation

After five minutes, start the second phase of your discussion about that same card. This time, talk to the question, "How would you want someone to respond to you if you made known to him the wish on the card?" Include in your discussion such things as what you would want a nurse to say to you; what material help to fulfill your wish you would be likely to expect (Don't worry about how *reasonable* your expectations are; be concerned only with what you want and need.); what you would want from other staff; what you would want from members of your family.

The discussion should reveal a number of alternative responses for those who nurse a patient bargaining for "just time enough" to fulfill his wishes. It should also provide ideas about what you might do to help him get what he needs. No nurse or health care person need assume the whole burden for responding effectively to the dying patient. Her function may often be to give messages to other people who are in a better position to fulfill the patient's needs. The importance of such a function cannot be minimized, since it is obvious that, if no one gets the message, no help can be forthcoming.

Discussion

In one class of physical therapists, a student related a personal experience she had with a dying patient bargaining for time. The patient—a man of about 65—was being attended by a private duty aide. As they sat and talked one day, he suddenly blurted out that he had treated his wife very badly during their marriage. His voice shook and tears came to his eyes as he told the aide that now it was too late to make amends. His wife had long since left him, married someone else, and was living thousands of miles away. There was no way—and no time—to atone for what he had done.

At first the aide was inclined to offer some superficial reassurance. It had happened a long time ago; the patient should forget about it and concentrate on the present. However, the nurse began to feel an undercurrent of anxiety herself. She felt helpless, quite certain that there was nothing she could do to fulfill this man's wish—to find some way for him to feel forgiven and at peace with himself.

Her supervising nurse admonished her for feeling uncomfortable, and pointed out that all she could do was to provide for the patient's physical-medical needs, and listen to him talk. But there *was* a way, the aide suddenly thought. She could take the message to the man's daughter—a devoted woman who visited him often and did everything she could to make him comfortable.

Eventually, the daughter convinced her father that at least part of the responsibility for the break up of his marriage was the attitude of his wife. She also convinced him that she and her brother and sister were not seriously hurt by the break up due to the love and understanding of their father and his constant efforts to make them feel wanted and secure.

Without the aide, the patient may never have had the opportunity to make his need known or to be reassured by his daughter. The aide, in effect, helped him bargain successfully.

Extending the Exericse

You may use the format of this exercise to examine other types of items for which people bargain. For example, you might make up a set of cards on which you have written—one to a card—the things you would want to make amends for before you die. These are generally sources of guilt for the individual: hurts you think you have done to others; neglects that you regret; lies that you would like to confess; love that you would like to express. Sometimes, the source of guilt lies hidden even from the patient. In this case, psychiatric help may be necessary to help the patient deal with it. Often, however, all the patient may require is the time and opportunity to make amends, and here is where the sensitive, accepting individual may be of direct assistance.

Another set of cards might be made up noting the people you would love to see again before you die. On these cards you would not write only the names of the people, since the others in your group will not be able to understand the significance of only a name. You would have to indicate also the relationship of that person to you. For example, you might write on one card: My childhood friend, Bess, whom I haven't seen for ten years. Or, on another card: My mother, whom I haven't seen in two years, since I left home.

Bargaining by the patient's family

It may be somewhat more difficult to help the patient's family who may also be engaged in bargaining—for more time, for less pain. Often, the bargaining is done privately, taking the form of appeals to God. Sometimes, people just wish—to themselves or to other members of the family—that things were not as they were.

If the family is religious, a clergyman may be alerted to the fact that workers in the field notice that families do go through this bargaining stage. Perhaps a tactful and sympathetic minister could more readily respond to signs if he knew what to look for.

Medical personnel should not assume that a minister of the same faith as the patient is always the ideal one to comfort people who face the imminent death of a loved one. As a matter of fact, the minister, no matter how concerned an individual he is, may be viewed by the family as intruding where he has no right to be. One such instance was the case of a man who was expected to die within a few days. The head nurse suggested to the minister who regularly visited the hospital that the family would probably appreciate a visit from him, since the man's illness had been sudden and the prognosis an unexpected and shocking development.

Though the minister was received politely, it was quite apparent that the family—grown children and their spouses, teen-age grandchildren, close relatives, all gathered at the man's home—were annoyed at the assumption that they either welcomed the intrusion of an outsider or that they would be interested in anything a minister could offer them. The nurse had assumed from the family's name that they were Jewish, and had made the further assumption that they were religious. The minister, a rabbi, came armed with the traditional comforts that the religion offered, but which meant nothing to this family. Actually, had the nurse been listening to her patient, she might have heard him "thank the *elements*" that his illness had not been transmitted to any of his progeny. And when he said, "If only nature would hold off until he could get over the shock of knowing he was going to die, he might be able to accept it eventually," it should have been clear that he was not bargaining with a God or any other traditional anthropomorphic symbol.

For those who are not religious, the nurse may initiate an open communication by telling a family member about some of the wishes expressed by the patient. This disclosure must first be approved by the patient. When a patient speaks to a nurse about his very personal thoughts, it must be assumed that he does so in confidence. The nurse who feels that he and his family can be helped by conveying his thoughts to them must first get his permision. Failure to secure such permission might very well put an end to the possibility of any future confidences—perhaps with disastrous results for the patient's welfare. Aside from this, however, to talk freely about what transpires between nurse and patient —no matter how beneficent the intent—is a violation of the patient's rights. Such talking can only be categorized as gossip, and cannot be justified professionally.

Clarifying one's own attitude toward bargaining (The zig-zag procedure)

Answer the following questions briefly. You may do this by yourself, just thinking about the answers, or as a group, by giving the answers aloud. Don't do any writing.*

1. Did you feel like coming to work (school) this morning?
2. If not, what did you wish you could do instead?
3. Do you have any reasonable expectation of being able to do what you'd like to do some day soon?
4. Do you ever expect to be able to do this?
5. What would you give to be able to do this now?
6. Can you imagine how it would be if you were sure you could never do what you have wanted to do—that you were going to die before you ever got the chance? How would you feel? What would you do? Would you attempt to make a deal with God, to give something in return for the opportunity to do what you wanted? Would you try to make a deal with your doctor? Your minister? Your nurse?
7. Is there someone you know who might be wishing for something before she dies? Can you help her make her wish known? Will you help her? When?

Discussion

This technique is designed to help people focus on a value area that they would like to clarify for themselves. The participants first respond to a number of rather innocuous questions ("the "zig" part of the procedure.) These questions draw one's attention because they deal with familiar experiences. They also encourage everyone to respond because the experiences are rather universally shared.

Responses to the first five questions are usually brief, casual and low-key, just as the questions are. The next questions (the "zag") on the key issue of dying usually catch the participants by surprise. They are forced to make a connection between a comfortable, familiar experience and a sharply poignant and unfamiliar one. The answers they give so casually take on new meaning in the serious context, and each participant is now

* The ideas for this and the next technique were found in Raths, Harmin, and Simon, *Values and Teaching* (Columbus, Ohio: Charles E. Merrill Publishing Company, 1966).

compelled to consider how far his expressed values will take him when he is confronted with the real issue.

Perhaps the crux of the matter here lies in the nature of the commitment that the individual is willing to make—the commitment to take action on his expressed values. If the participant is inclined to bargain for what he wants and needs, is he willing to accept this behavior in other people? Is he ready to encourage them to bargain overtly if he only suspects that they are doing so secretly? Or does he himself engage in this behavior but is unwilling to admit that it is "respectable" behavior, and that he has a role in reassuring people of its respectability?

Medical personnel might consider that they are often inclined to avoid noticing bargaining behavior, partly because they have some anxiety about not being able to fulfill a patient's wishes. Can it be that another reason for the avoidance is that the behavior is considered somewhat immature, childish, involved in fantasy, and so inappropriate for adults? Then where do our values really lie when we engage in behavior clandestinely and permit neither ourselves nor others to reveal the need for it?

Devil's advocate

Here is a point of view about bargaining in the face of death. Someone might read it aloud to the group and then the group can examine it, agreeing, disagreeing, examining various alternatives and the consequences of those alternatives. When you have finished your discussion, you should be pretty clear about how you feel about bargaining.

It is ridiculous to believe for a moment that one can prevent or postpone the inevitable.. There is no point in trying to cajole the fates into granting one more day, one more opportunity, one more pain-free moment. Even if there is a God, why would anyone in his right mind believe that He would be bothered to change one person's destiny when so many millions in the world continue to suffer and die?

Once a medical diagnosis has been made, there is nothing a patient can do except to submit to whatever treatment is available for decreasing his discomfort and to make as little fuss as possible. If there were other things that could be done, the patient would not have to bargain for them.

Bargaining makes everyone uncomfortable, because the medical staff is usually helpless to do anything about fulfilling the patient's—or his family's—wishes. The more uncomfortable people feel, the less able they are to attend to the medical aspects of care. So, in the end, the patient is the one who loses if he or his family persist in such foolish behavior.

Death is not a punishment for being "bad," in the way a child is punished by a parent. We must all die some day, and it is not in our power to postpone that day. Making promises that will probably never be kept is just an exercise in futility. No professional should ever take these promises seriously.

Confronted with such an extreme statement, it is almost impossible for people to remain silent. In the rush to refute, argue, and even agree, it is not only likely that a person will clarify his own stand on the issue, but he also will make public commitment to certain values. Once he has made public his point of view, he is more likely to act on it, especially when those who heard him take a stand are the same people who work side by side with him.

Of course, the one who takes the Devil's Advocate position should be given the opportunity to make it perfectly clear that the position is not really his own, that he was just playing a role for purposes of discussion.

chapter six

———◄◦►———

Grieving

Identifying the stage

Kübler-Ross identifies grieving as the fourth stage in the dying process. The patient at this time enters a period of behavior similar to the behavior of people who are losing someone they love. Kavenaugh *(Facing Death)* suggests that the stages of dying as described by Kübler-Ross are very similar to the stages of grieving. Perhaps the dying process is, in reality, a process of grieving—grieving for the ultimate loss, the loss of oneself. Though we generally think of those who grieve as the *family* of the patient, the patient certainly also has basis for grief. He faces the loss of not one, but *all* his loved ones. And he faces also loss of himself and all the things that are important to him.

In our society, different values are assigned to different manifestations of grief. Our valuing criteria also are adjusted for different ages and sexes. Consequently, we see some behaviors as appropriate and desirable, and so deserving of sympathetic and empathic responses. Other behaviors we reject as unworthy, thus also rejecting the person who engages in this behavior.

For example, as a society we abhor "self-pity." The term "self-pity" causes us to form images of weak-willed creatures deserving the contempt of those who are strong and courageous. Nobody wants to be accused of self-pity, though it is a wonder how we can ever lend ourselves to pitying others when we are so hard on ourselves. We are, after all, pitying the sadness of the entire human condition. Why can't we be sad to know that we are going to die? Why shouldn't we grieve about the pain and suffering to which we are heir?

Many people associate the grieving behavior of a dying patient with self-pity. Not only do we thereby reassert our own superiority over the one who is displaying the wrong kind of behavior, but we also absolve ourselves from the necessity for making caring and helping responses. This is a secondary gain that serves to remove us from a situation that may cause us great discomfort. If the grieving person doesn't deserve our help, we can leave him to his blubbering and go on to more deserving recipients of our ministrations.

Actually, a man has the right to cry for himself when he is facing the loss of everything he knows and loves. He has a right to cry about the work he will leave unfinished, the things he will never get to do. Not only is it his right, but it is also quite reasonable for him to do so. The chances are that if you don't see evidences in his behavior that he is grieving, he is merely managing to keep it hidden from other people. Before we commend him for his stoicism, we ought to conjecture about his reasons for hiding his grief. Is he consciously pretending not to grieve so that he may present to the people around him the image of a person they are more likely to accept? How much energy and suffering is going into maintaining this façade? Would it be a great relief to him to grieve openly, confident that the grieving will be accepted?

Does the man hide his grief because he needs the show of calm if he is to continue to function reasonably? Does he make a choice to do his grieving privately, just as he has done all his life, because his own public grief would be too frightening for him?

Is he reluctant to admit grief so that he may maintain the stereotype of the man in our society: Men don't cry; only women do? Does he need reassurance that the stereotype is just that: a lie?

Grieving may be done in secret for still another reason. Patients who are lied to about their imminent death are prevented from grieving normally. They often feel they must hide their grief from those around them, and thus they are condemned to isolation and loneliness at a time when they desperately need consolation. For that consolation is substituted hollow cheerfulness and bewildering and suffocating pampering.

The families that withhold their consolation at this time are more fortunate than the patient. They, at least, are able to grieve with each other. The patient can only see the red eyes, hear the empty reassurances and suffer his grief alone, unless he is able to find some single person— a nurse, an aide, the patient in the next bed—who will permit him to cry aloud.

An Exercise in Responding to Grief

Both dying patients and their families need similar kinds of help to ease them through the period of grief to a point of acceptance of death. What Kübler-Ross identifies as the process of dying for the patient, Kavanaugh describes as the process of grieving for the patient's family. Both the family and the person dying seem to pass through similar stages. Kübler-Ross' fourth stage of dying—depression—is much like the guilt and the sense of loneliness and loss that is a part of Kavanaugh's description of grief. Thus, exercises designed to learn how to interact with a dying patient may also be useful to learn how to interact with someone who is grieving for a dying person. The following exercise may be useful in practicing skills for interacting with dying people and people who are grieving for a loved one.

Before you have a chance to read Kavanaugh or anyone else on the subject of grief, try this exercise with the other members of your group. Make up a set of cards with one of the following items on each card. (Do not write the numbers on the cards; they are merely keys to the discussion that follows the game.)

(1) laughter
(1) fainting
(1) "No! No! It's not possible!"
(1) "Doctors don't know everything! Couldn't they be wrong?"

(2) doesn't prepare meals for her young children
(2) doesn't eat
(2) look of non-recognition
(2) "Why did it have to happen?"
(2) insists on taking the children to the movies
(2) "Are you sure?"

(3) screaming
(3) breaking valuable objects
(3) running away
(3) locking one's self in a room
(3) has hysterics
(3) begins to drink
(3) gets into the car and prepares to drive away

(1,2,3) "I can't go on living without her! I want to die, too."
(1,2,3) crying uncontrollably

(1,2,3) "We'll take him to the Mayo Clinic!"

(1,2,3) tearing her hair

(1,2,3) "I'll kill myself! I'll jump out the window!"

(1,2,3) "They said they could cure him! They promised it wouldn't be long before they found a cure!"

(1,2,3) "He's still breathing! Look! He's still breathing!"

(1,2,3) look of confusion, as if he doesn't understand what you're saying

(1,2,3) talks and talks and talks—about his childhood, the progress of the illness, all he's done for the patient, what he must do now, questions about what will happen to him, etc, etc. . . .

(3) "How could he do this to me? I hate him! I hate him!"

(3) "Now he's out of it! He's free! And what about me? What am I supposed to do now?"

(3) "I'm so scared! I'm so scared!" Sits doubled over, rocking back and forth obviously terror-stricken.

(3) tight-lipped silence. But his face looks very angry.

(3) walks out on the graveside eulogy: "Who the hell is *he* to say such things. He didn't know her! He doesn't care about her! What does he know about how I feel?"

(4) "It was all my fault. I knew he was overworking!"

(4) "I left home! I broke her heart!"

(4) "He always wanted me to go into business with him. How could I have been so selfish?"

(4) "I was always nagging him about money. I know now how unimportant money is!"

(4) "We should have spent more time together. I was always saying the children came first."

(4) "I didn't care enough. I never cared enough!"

(4) "He was dying and I was out having a good time!"

(4) "I should have listened to him. I should have spent more time listening to him!"

(4) "It's my fault—all my fault! There's something wrong in me. That's why he's going to die!"

(5) Several months after the daughter has died, the parents are very sad and depressed. Feel very lonely. Feel an overwhelming sense of loss.

(5) Woman, five months after the death of her husband, is planning to marry again.

(5) Man, several months after the death of his child, is urging his wife to adopt another child.

(6) "I feel drained. All I can think of is that I don't have to go to the

hospital night after night. I can relax after work—and just watch television."

(6) "It was so hard to sit there beside his bed all those hours and not be able to think of anything to say."

(6) "I was tired all the time. It was so hard to keep going."

(6) "She's better off dead. Nobody could stand to see her suffer any more."

(7) "Let's go out to dinner and a show. It's been a long time since we did that."

(7) "Sorry I keep missing your calls; I've met some people and we've been visiting."

Check to see that you have a set of forty-nine cards, each containing one of the above examples of behavior. Shuffle the cards well. Now, sit in a small circle of eight or nine people and put the set of cards in the middle. One person at a time should pick a card and describe the behavior written on it, attributing the behavior to someone close to a patient of his who has just died or who has just been given a diagnosis of a terminal illness.

For example, take the first item on the list, *laughter.* The person who picks that card might say, "My patient's daughter, a twenty-five-year-old woman, began to laugh when the doctor told her that her father was going to die. The doctor just turned on his heel and walked out, and I was left with her. What could I do in such a situation?"

The people in the group may give suggestions about helping the daughter. They should also say what one absolutely should not do in the situation. However, the one who presented the incident must make the final decision about how he would help his patient's daughter. He writes down his decision and puts it away for future reference, without telling anyone what he has written.

When a number of cards have been discussed, read the rest of the section. It may be useful to keep in mind what the group thought was helpful and your own final decision.

Discussion

The listed behaviors in the above exercise are identified by numbers 1 through 7, corresponding to Kavanaugh's stages of grieving:*

1. shock
2. disorganization

* Kavanaugh, *Facing Dealth,* pp. 107, ff.

3. volatile emotions
4. guilt
5. loss and loneliness
6. relief
7. re-establishment

Often, both outsiders and other grieving persons do not recognize the behaviors in the exercise as characteristic of grieving, because they view grief as a stereotypic presentation of sadness, tears, and withdrawal from pleasure. Consequently, they may respond to dissimilar behaviors with disapproval and rejection at the very time the grieving person most desperately needs acceptance.

For example, the young son who laughs uncontrollably when he is told that his father has just died does not need someone to admonish him for his inappropriate behavior—no matter how gentle the scolding. It is easy enough for us to deal with fainting—administering the conventional remedies obviously fills the immediate need. But, even more, fainting is a conventionally *appropriate* response to shocking news. We can even permit a man to faint under such conditions. But his laughter in itself may be shocking, and it is difficult to look beneath it to the feeling of shock that caused it. Just as a fainting person may be quickly revived by stimulants, the laughing person may also be quickly revived by having his hand lovingly held and by repeating, "It's all right, it's all right," in a low, reassuring voice.

Similarly, the person who asks, "Couldn't the doctors be wrong?" is really not asking for information at that moment. The chances are that he would not be able to assimilate a rational answer. What he is crying out is more a statement of disbelief than a search for answers. His "It's not possible!" is a similar kind of denial, and a nurse's mere presence is more comforting than trying to institute "sensible" communication.

As in so much purposive, conscious behavior, we have a tendency to emphasize the rational. It is almost as if we are forever trying to prove to ourselves that we are, above all, clear-thinking, intelligent, *objective* human beings, only minimally motivated by emotion. Whatever help we stand prepared to offer is help based on "common sense," "cool-headedness," "professionalism." (Professionalism is to be equated with knowledge, skill, and *no* emotional involvement.)

The almost universal need to see ourselves as more intellectual than emotional may cause us to commit serious errors in the helping relationship. For example, we may feel impelled to urge grieving people to "get hold" of themselves. We want them to resume their customary life routines in the belief that such routine will help them recover more quickly from their loss. The result of this urging and pushing is likely, in the beginning, to be completely futile; and a little later, to be a destructive interference with the grieving process. At first, during the period of disorganization, grieving people may not even hear the urgings to keep going. They may not even recognize the speaker or recall his name. When they finally do make sense of the words, they may interpret them as a mandate to hide their grief and put on a mask of equanimity for the world. If they succeed in doing this, then the unfinished grieving may forever afterward drain off energy and serenity and prevent optimum adjustment to loss.

The period of disorganization may be characterized by crying. It is important to permit men to cry as well as women. Or the person may talk endlessly about the past and the lost one. It is better to let this go on without interruption. The person who wants to help need only be there to listen and to murmur an occasional reassurance.

Some grieving behavior rises from a feeling of disorganization. Uncharacteristic behavior of a grieving person should not be a reason for reprimanding. The woman who does not prepare meals for her children or does not eat when meals are prepared by others, the father who insists on taking his children to the movies to cheer them on the afternoon their mother died—these people need gentleness and understanding, not a scolding.

Threats of suicide from a grieving person can often call forth severe disapproval. Such threats come from shock, anger and fear, and need loving responses rather than disapproval. Hugging, reassuring words, mere physical presence of a caring friend can help a person through this. (It has been observed that excessive and prolonged mourning of a child, for example, can actually precipitate the suicide of another child in the family. The child who is forgotten—even temporarily—and whose own mourning is not dealt with—may begin to believe that the only way he can obtain his parents' love is by dying. This feeling, combined with feelings of guilt, anger, and other unresolved emotions of grieving, may cause him to take his own life.)

Certainly, the bereaved person should not make major decisions during his period of disorganization. His family, and the medical staff, should help him with decisions yet not force him into a decision he may later regret. Most decisions can probably be delayed a day or two until the grieving person can face reality. The more loving and accepting that world is, the more likely it is that his return will be sooner rather than later.

After the period of disorganization, growing realization of loss may result in hysteria, screaming, breaking objects, or the need to run or hide. A bereaved person needs to feel free to be himself and not feel compelled to put on an act that keeps the screaming inside. Only with this freedom to be himself can he pass through his mourning and resume his normal life. Interference with the process by forcing him to go through the motions of "acceptable" behavior may make those around him feel more comfortable; yet, this person may be left with a residue of unfinished mourning for the rest of his life.

Especially uncomfortable for friends and other bystanders are the outbursts of anger directed against the one who has died. "How could he do this to me?! I hate him! I hate him!" can be a shocking statement for friends to hear from a newly-bereaved wife. She may be crying out of her fear of being alone and her helplessness in the face of inexorable loss. Her husband's death becomes another instance of his neglect, of leaving her to cope with a problem child or a domestic calamity. Friends need to feel the confusion and hurt behind the outburst and offer love instead of disapproval.

Because one "ought not" to feel this way, the tendency is to quiet the grieving person. Some people give reasons why the dead did or did not do what the bereaved is now resenting. The physician gives sedatives and tranquilizers.

Of course, the most idyllic of human relationships have times of anger and resentment. To suppress such feelings so that we may perpetuate the fiction that the dead person was perfect and perfectly loved is to perpetuate a pretense that can interfere with a real appreciation of the relationship between the bereaved and the dead.

Because the bereaved may prefer to deny any deviation from some ideal of perfection in his close relationship, the imperfections of reality inevitably come back to haunt him. This is especially true when death removes the last possibility that the relationship can ever be improved. The guilt needs to be expressed and the listener should not judge. Just forgive, so that the bereaved may finally feel free to forgive himself.

Kübler-Ross identifies in the fourth stage of the dying process a reactive depression that contains elements of Kavanaugh's guilt. Here the dying patient reacts to such practical concerns as small children who will be left without a parent, or families who will be left without a source of income. He and his family can use practical help in solving these problems. Though medical personnel are generally not the ones to offer such help, they can inform individuals of agencies whose function is to provide such assistance. It is not too far-fetched to expect the nurse in today's bureaucratized, agency-oriented society to become familiar with the varieties of assistance that are available in the hospital community. She cannot function in the hospital believing it is an isolated society whose concerns begin and end at the building boundaries. The day she finds herself assigned to a "satellite" clinic in the heart of an urban community, she may realize with dismay how important it is to know what is happening in her community.

Not only does the patient who feels guilty need practical help, but also he can benefit from reassurance that he is not at fault. It is commendable that the dying patient makes plans to fulfill his obligations. Surely this is appreciated by his family! The nurse may wish to draw the family members into a discussion to let them hear the patient's expressions of guilt so that they may join in the protestations with love and reassurance.

Also in Kübler-Ross' fourth stage of dying is what she terms preparatory depression. This stage sounds similar to Kavanaugh's fifth stage of loss and loneliness. Here the dying person prepares himself for the loss of the whole world. Reassurance is no help to him now. He may need opportunity to express his feelings to someone who is willing to just listen silently or touch him gently. He is sad; he needs someone who will be near him and accept his sadness.

As time goes on, sadness and a sense of loss also become the dominant mood of those who are grieving for a loved one who has died. They feel a great emptiness, and without the continuing presence of people who care, can impulsively fill that emptiness in a way they might soon regret. It is during this time, when consolers may have returned to the business of their own lives and are assuming that their grieving friend has done the same, that their friend needs them.

Gradually, the griever is able to admit to himself—and hopefully to good friends who have, by their frequent presence, made it clear that they are there to listen, to help, and to accept without judging—that it is a relief to be free of the suffering, to be free to do other things besides sit in the hospital day after day, to be free of waiting for good news and fearing bad news. The good friends should not add to the remnants of guilt and shame that accompany the relief; they should accept the hesitant expressions of relief as natural and acceptable.

Slowly the "might-have-beens" and "why didn't I's" fade into the background, and the griever is able to pick up the threads of his life again. Old friends may now be a little too eager to push him into new experiences and new relationships, when what he wants are some of the old, comfortable diversions. Friends may continue to give comfort and emphasize sadness, when he is trying to overcome this sadness. Perhaps at this time, some new friends who do not view him as a bereaved person are more comfortable to be with. This does not mean that he should—or wants to—drop the friends who stayed with him while he mourned. It merely suggests that this may be a time to enlarge his circle of associates.

The preceding discussion does not present all the data being accumulated about the mourning process. For this there is a growing body of literature that is readily accessible. The discussion merely highlights the observable aspects of the behavior of a grieving person with an eye to considering and practicing appropriate helping responses as each aspect becomes apparent to the observer.

Lest the thought occurs to you, there is nothing cold-blooded or un-feeling about a deliberate attempt to identify grieving behavior and to practice helping. You may think that there is something more honest and warm about spontaneity in the face of intense emotion. However, when that spontaneity arises out of lack of experience, lack of knowledge, and personal discomfort, it can merely add to the mourner's burden of grief. It seems rather hard to leave your learning about how to respond to grief to one of the most primitive of learning processes—trial and error. While we are learning, the ones who need our help are a prey to each one of our attempts that results in hurt rather than help.

This does not mean that we can eliminate all error from our attempts to help by engaging in exercises in an educational situation. However, there is no doubt that the margin for error in our choices of appropriate behavior can be substantially reduced by this kind of reflection and practice. If the validity of this principle were not already clearly estab-lished, what justification would we have for any kind of institutional education? We would do better by just letting people grow up trying everything and learning only by the results of their trials. If we did this, each generation would need to invent the wheel all over again, relive the errors of his ancestors, and have use only of that knowledge that he himself was able to accumulate by direct experience. We can be much more efficient than this about learning by selecting a variety of experi-ences that can make us more effective when we are faced with the neces-sity for functioning in a real situation.

In thinking about this discussion, have you changed your mind about any of your methods to help grieving people? Have you found a bias in your decisions that seems to reflect some aspect of your own personality, rather than the needs of the griever? For example: Do you believe that expressing strong emotions should be done in private? Are you impatient with people who seem to give up control over their own lives—even if they do so only temporarily? Do you prefer that men behave one way in the face of adversity, and women another? Are you quick to give advice when a person cannot solve his problems? Do you so firmly believe in the comforts of your religion that you insist that others be similarly comforted, even though they have different religious beliefs, or no beliefs at all?

If you can answer yes to any of these questions, perhaps you ought to re-examine your approach to helping those who grieve. If you feel that none of these apply to you, perhaps you ought to ask your classmates for help in evaluating your helping decisions. It is possible that you are too personally committed to see the relationship between your decisions and your own needs.

chapter seven

———————◀◆▶———————

Acceptance

Identifying the stage

"If a patient has had enough time . . . and has been given some help in working through the previously described stages, he will reach a stage during which he is neither depressed nor angry . . . and he will contemplate his coming end with a certain degree of quiet expectation." *

Following are descriptions of dying and grieving people who seem to have reached the stage of acceptance. After each description are questions designed to help you pinpoint some of the problems experienced by hospital personnel and family members who do not recognize or understand the patient's feelings.

Ms. Linton

Jim Smith, the charge nurse on the unit, was surprised to see Judy Linton crying bitterly on the sofa in the sitting room. Every time he had seen her since her mother's admission to the hospital three weeks ago she had been calm. She seemed to have accepted the fact that her mother was very ill and was not expected to recover. Judy had spoken freely to him about the long year of treatment and remissions and had revealed own

———

* Kübler-Ross, *On Death and Dying*, p. 112.

feelings of frustration and anger when she realized that someone as young as her mother could not be helped by the doctors. She had gone through a time when she could not seem to stop crying. But in time she was able to talk calmly with her mother, responding honestly to questions about her own future and reassuring her mother that she was provided for and would be all right.

Now here she was, seemingly thrust back into anguish, unable to control her crying when Jim sat down beside her and asked her what was the matter.

Finally, her crying subsided somewhat and she was able to speak between long, shaky sobs. Her mother, she said, had turned away from her. She no longer cared about her. "Is it something I've done—or not done?" she asked. "Why is she angry with me? What's happened?"

"Why do you think she's angry with you?" Jim asked. "Did she say something to make you think that?"

"N-no. It was nothing she said, exactly. I just sort of get the feeling that she doesn't want me to visit her any more."

"Can you tell me more about it? Did she do something that made you feel that way?"

"Oh . . . I don't know. . . . She doesn't care what happens to me." Judy burst into tears again and, for the moment, Jim only patted her back and made vague, reassuring sounds until she was able to talk with him again.

Questions for Discussion

1. What specific behaviors do you think Judy saw that made her feel her mother no longer cared about her?
2. How do you account for Judy's apparent regression to an earlier stage of grief?
3. What was Jim's objective in asking questions?
4. What questions do you think he will ask her when she stops crying? What will be gained by asking them?
5. Is there something you think Jim Smith should tell Judy? What is it and what would it accomplish?

Mr. Chaco

Mr. Chaco has been unable to admit to his wife and son that he now knows he is going to die shortly—that he has known it for weeks. They are so determinedly cheerful and optimistic, that he sometimes finds it hard to believe that they, too, know his end is very near.

One day, exhausted not only by his illness but also by his pretense, he made an attempt to say something to his family, "Please," he ventured, interrupting a glowing account of a vacation they would all take as soon as he was out of the hospital. "Please, don't do this to us. I'm so tired. Let me sleep. Let me sleep forever."

"What are you saying!" His wife almost screamed her protest. "Of course you're tired; you've been sick. Take a nap now, and we'll be right outside waiting for you. We have to finalize our plans. You'll have to let us know what you want us to pack for you. What is it going to be, Bill? Golf, or just relaxing on the beach?"

Mr. Chaco looked at his wife a moment. When he turned to his son, the young man smiled at him brightly. Finally, he sighed and turned on his side. He closed his eyes and dozed off, gently closing a door on his wife and son.

Questions for Discussion

1. What behavioral clues do you have that Mr. Chaco has reached the point of accepting his imminent death?
2. At what stage of grief are his wife and son?
3. Apparently, some member or members of the medical staff have been involved in the psychological process of Mr. Chaco's dying. What do you think they have been doing and saying?
4. Do you think medical personnel have also been involved in the process of the family's grief? What evidence do you have of such involvement —or lack of involvement?

John Blair

"Dr. Morton, I must speak to you!" Mrs. Blair looked very troubled. Although Ralph Morton was on his way to an important meeting, he felt obliged to stop and speak to his patient's wife.

"What's the matter, Mrs. Blair? Let's sit down here." He led her into the waiting room.

"Doctor, it's John. Something terrible has happened to him!"

He looked at her oddly. What in the world was the woman talking about? He had himself told her that her husband was not expected to survive the month. Was she only now realizing what she had heard a week ago?

"Tell me, Mrs. Blair. What is it you think has happened?"

"I think John is losing his mind!" Her eyes opened wide in fear and incredulity. Her hand went up to her mouth and her head shook back and forth as if to deny what she herself had just said.

For a moment Dr. Morton was confused. Nothing in John Blair's condition should cause behavior so bizarre that his wife might think he had lost his mind. Besides, he'd seen his patient an hour ago, and he had seemed quite calm—at peace with himself and the world.

"Doctor," the woman went on. "He must be insane! He's happy that he's going to die. He actually wants to die! You must do something! You've got to snap him out of it! You've got to help him!"

Questions for Discussion

1. Why do you think Mrs. Blair thought her husband was happy about his death?
2. How can you explain the apparent contradiction between Dr. Morton's view of Mr. Blair's behavior and Mrs. Blair's perception of that same behavior?
3. Is there something that can be said or done that would help Mrs. Blair evaluate her husband's behavior more realistically?
4. Do you think there is something that might be said to the patient which would facilitate communication between himself and his wife?

Mrs. Traymore

Mrs. Traymore is an old woman who has a large family—children, adult grandchildren, and several great-grandchildren. She has always been an active, talkative woman, involved in every facet of her family's life. She could never be characterized as a quiet woman.

Just as she has always squarely and courageously faced the good and bad in her own and her family's circumstances, she has quickly come to terms with the fact of her own dying. Similarly, her family, after the initial shock of learning of their matriarch's fatal illness, went through a period of anger and noisy grieving before they began to visit the hospital regularly, bringing treats, laughing and talking among themselves, and keeping the old woman abreast of the many family happenings.

Slowly they began to realize that Mrs. Traymore was not participating in the noise and discussion. Most of the time she seemed far away from them and looked extremely tired.

After a family conclave, they concluded that it would be better for the patient if they stayed out of her room and let her rest quietly. Occasionally, one of them would look in, see her lying there quietly, and close the door without going in. From being the center of what often looked to outsiders like commotion, Mrs. Traymore was now virtually alone.

One day, Ms. Green, the nurse on the floor, came into the room and found her patient extremely depressed. "They're all tired of waiting for me to die," she said. "I thought they cared about me."

Questions for Discussion

1. Although Mrs. Traymore could no longer actually participate in the life of her family, what kind of interaction did she still need?
2. What needs of the family might have been provided for by their decision to withdraw from the company of the patient?
3. What benefit could the members of the family have derived from changing their behavior with Mrs. Traymore instead of stopping their visits?
4. Specifically, what could Ms. Green do to help both Mrs. Traymore and her family?

Jimmy MacKlin

Mrs. MacKlin, Jimmy's mother, was furious at Ms. Hamilton, the nurse assigned to care for Jimmy. She had complained to the charge nurse and the doctor, and was threatening to see the director of the hospital and insist that Ms. Hamilton be fired.

When she was calm for a moment, Ms. Johnson, the charge nurse, persuaded her to sit down and accept a glass of water. Ms. Johnson sat down facing her. "What did Ms. Hamilton do that made you so angry?" Ms. Johnson asked her.

"What did she do!" Mrs. MacKlin was still seething with anger. "What did she do! I caught her telling Jimmy he was going to die! The nerve of that woman—saying a thing like that to a child! And it's not true, anyway! He's getting better! He's been much better the last few days. Anyone can see he's getting better!"

Ms. Johnson bit her lip. Jimmy was twenty-four-years-old. He had demanded and received a full account of his condition, and he knew that he would never leave the hospital again. His mother had naturally been distraught. At the height of her grief when she cried continually, she saw her son become calm, peaceful, and apparently unconcerned about his illness.

What Mrs. MacKlin did not know was that while she was immersed in her grief, the staff of the hospital had rallied around her son. They had spent time with him around the clock, listening to him, helping him, accepting his feelings, and sharing their own. Now Jimmy was finished with fear and despair, and most of his sadness was for his grieving mother.

Mrs. MacKln's rage was precipitated when she walked unexpectedly into her son's room and heard him say to Ms. Hamilton, "I don't want to die, but I'm not afraid anymore. Thanks to you and everybody here."

Questions for Discussion

1. Why did Mrs. MacKlin think her son was recovering?
2. How do you account for the intensity of her anger against Ms. Hamilton whom she had seen care lovingly for her son for weeks?
3. Do you think Mrs. MacKlin would have believed Ms. Johnson if she were told that Jimmy was not recovering, and had accepted the fact of his dying?
4. Is there anything that could have been done to help the mother whose son was dying?

Philip Tryon

Ellen Casey's mother had died when she was sixteen and her brother Philip was thirteen. She had assumed the responsibility of managing their home, cooking meals for her brother and father, and making sure that her brother went to school regularly and kept out of trouble. In spite of her efforts, Philip quit school and left home when he was fourteen, hitchhiking around the country until he could no longer manage. Half sick, hungry, and two-thousand miles from home, he had enlisted in the army. In the ensuing twenty years he had been seriously wounded and had contracted liver disease. Ellen always felt guilty because she had not made their home satisfying enough for him to stay.

Now Philip was dying, and Ellen spent every waking hour at his bedside, fussing over him, and harassing hospital personnel in her belief that she was helping him to recover. Actually, Philip was a man who had lived a full life and a good one and had no feeling of things left undone. He had accepted his doctor's word that everything possible had been done.

Ellen's husband, after watching her behavior one afternoon in the hospital, and seeing the troubled look on Philip's face, tries to convince her that she ought to take the evening off. He offers to take her to dinner and to the movies. She is outraged at the suggestion. "How can you even think I'd go out to have a good time when Philip is here? I know he's not *your* brother, but you could have some feeling for someone who is d-d-d. . . ."

"Ellen, Philip wants you to go on with your life. He doesn't want you fussing over him. He's tired. He needs time to himself—time to rest."

"You're wrong. He needs me. He's going to be all right. He needs me."

"He needs you to sit quietly and hold his hand once in a while. He doesn't need all this pulling and pushing. He has accepted what's happening; don't you understand?"

She pulls away from him in anger. "You don't care about him! You don't care the way I do! Leave me alone! Let me go to him!"

Questions for Discussion

1. Who do you think is right about what Philip needs: Ellen or her husband?
2. Why does Ellen seem to be so sure that her brother will recover?
3. Ellen cannot, for a moment, stop thinking about her brother's fatal illness. Do you think the same is true of Philip, that he thinks only of the fact that he is dying?
4. What can be done—and by whom—to make Ellen aware of the reality of her brother's condition?

Emory Smith

Emory Smith learned several weeks ago that he has a fatal illness. The illness is not incapacitating. Though he must return to the hospital regularly for treatments, he is able, between treatments, to live a relatively normal life. He has decided to spend what time he has left talking with other people who do not have long to live. He also has initiated a vigorous campaign to raise money for research into the causes of his illness.

In public, he speaks candidly about his imminent death, but he likes to say that he is not dying—he is "still living." Although the people in the community admire and praise him, Smith's wife feels only anger and frustration. She is firmly convinced that he refuses to believe he is dying. She wants him to spend his time resting—and in the company of his family. Instead, she feels he is never home, and that his strength is being squandered for strangers.

Questions for Discussion

1. Is Emory Smith engaging in denial, or has he come to terms with his death? (What behavioral cues lead you to your decision?)
2. Is it possible to reconcile the needs of Mr. Smith and his wife, or are they diametrically opposed?
3. How do you think the medical staff who care for Mr. Smith feel about his activities? What role do they have in reconciling the needs of husband and wife?

Role-playing

You may feel that discussing the questions in each case does not always result in clear-cut alternatives for helping the people involved. If you assume the roles of patient, family members, doctor and nurse, and act out the central conflict, you may find answers that your discussion did not reveal. In role-playing, you may more easily see the consequences of different courses of action. Thus, if you are faced with a similar situation one day, you may be better prepared to avoid undesirable consequences.

Reading about the experiences of physicians and nurses who have worked with the dying is valuable for building a foundation of information about behavior. We can, through such reading, also respond with compassion to the feelings of others. Talking with each other helps us take another step toward empathy and understanding, as we recount our experiences and express our feelings.

Role-playing brings us as close to the living experience as we can come and still be safe. Errors we make as role-players are never a matter of life and death. Consequences are always revocable. We also have the opportunity to take on roles and practice behaviors we never thought we could. By role-playing, we may learn to face the real situation with greater confidence and composure than we would with a preparation only of lectures and readings.

section three

Trajectories of Dying

chapter eight

———◄●●►———

The Social-Psychological Significance of the Dying Trajectory

The dying trajectory defined

"How a doctor, a nurse, or a family member defines a dying trajectory becomes the basis for his or her behavior in connection with treating and handling the patient" (Glaser and Strauss, *Time for Dying*). The trajectory—or course of the patient's dying—may be speedy or slow; it may be a surprise, as when a patient who is expected to recover suddenly dies; it may be expected, as when a patient with cancer lingers for a long time. It may be appropriate, as when an old person dies, or inappropriate, as when a child dies.

A patient's dying trajectory is not the actual course of his dying, but rather a perceived course. This perception is inevitably a function of the knowledge, experiences, feelings, and beliefs of the medical staff. Since, according to a number of observers in the field, doctors do not usually communicate their perception of a patient's trajectory to the nurses, and since nurses consequently depend on the reading of their own cues to determine a patient's dying trajectory, a patient's hospital experience can be determined, not only by the nature of the medical problem, but also, apparently, by the social and idiosyncratic attitudes of the staff. Since the professional schedule of work as well as personal interaction is based on how long the patient is expected to live and the way he is expected to live, hospital personnel must develop an awareness of the psychological

processes known as stereotypic thinking, selective perception, and prejudice, as they operate in determining a dying trajectory.

Stereotypic thinking

Efficient thinking is at least partly dependent upon the ability of the
thinker to generalize from significant cues. Thus, when we see someone
on the hospital floor carrying a small black bag and a stethoscope, and
asking for a patient's chart, we can safely assume that he is a physician.
(There is, of course, always a margin of potential error in any kind of
generalization; occasionally an imposter takes advantage of our need to
generalize, and he assumes the significant cues to fool us.) However, often
we learn to generalize from cues that are not relevant. For example, a
white person may see someone with dark skin and conclude that he is a
criminal. A man who sees a woman's car break down may assume that,
because she is a woman, she will be helpless to repair the trouble herself.

To conclude from certain cues that we know what a person is like is
to stereotype that person. We expect women to express their feelings of
fear and sadness and men to be stoic. We frequently assume that every
old person we meet is childish and stubborn and that, if he is ill or very
old, he is finished with life. We see children laughing and playing and
believe they are free from worry and care. We extend our belief to feel
that we can easily keep children from the knowledge of the sadness and
tragedy of life. (Actually, all we do is cut off communication between
children and ourselves, because children *do* worry, *do* know about death,
and *do* have fears and anxieties that they learn to keep from *us*.)

Below is an exercise in stereotypic thinking. After responding to the
exercise, you may wish to discuss your feelings with the group. You may
be surprised to discover how similar your responses are.

What cues do you use?

Read each situation below and make a list of the significant information
on which you would base your relationship with the patient and the
patient's family. Next to each item of information, you should note such
pertinent observations as:

This symptom doesn't seem serious; the chances are that the patient
will be able to receive treatment in the doctor's office.

This person sounds interesting; I'd like to know what he/she does for
a living.

This symptom probably means cancer; it doesn't look good.

This patient is an unpleasant man; I'll just try to stay away from him as much as possible.

After you have done this with all four situations, you might like to read the discussion that follows and see how your conclusions match up with what actually happened in each case.

SITUATION #1: A man of about thirty-five is admitted to the hospital. He appears strong and healthy, but he has been suffering recurrent urinary infections, which, though mild, are annoying. His doctor has suggested that the source of infection needs to be pinpointed. He is a pleasant man, smiling and easy-going. He rarely rings for help, preferring to attend to his own needs. He has many visitors—mostly people of his own age—and his room is always bursting with laughter and conversation.

SITUATION #2: Ms. Milton is unconsolable. She has been crying ever since her doctor told her that she would have to have a hysterectomy. Although she is twenty-eight and the mother of a six-year-old and a four-year-old, she had been planning to have another child with her second husband. (Both of her children by the first husband were born with severe physical deformities.)

Ms. Milton has not yet re-married, but she and her fiancé have been seeing each other for about three months. Actually, they have been living together for most of that time.

Though Ms. Milton's problem has been diagnosed as a possible tumor, the doctors do not think it is malignant. Naturally, even the remote possibility that it might be also disturbs her.

Ms. Milton is white.

SITUATION #3: Mr. Lupton will probably die in a few days. Although the doctor has not mentioned this to anyone, including Mr. Lupton, the nurses have agreed that he does not have much time. This is his third admission to the hospital in the past year, and they can see that his condition has significantly deteriorated.

Mr. Lupton is very irritable and angry most of the time. He shouts at everyone and criticizes the things they do for him. His manner causes nervous responses which also infuriate him: everyone keeps dropping things, hypodermic syringes miss their mark, nurses stutter in response to his questions and thus seem evasive and uncommunicative.

Even Mr. Lupton's wife and children are targets for his anger. Almost every visiting hour, one of them leaves his room in tears. None of the staff knows if the family is aware of his imminent death. No one has broached the subject with them.

SITUATION #4: Ms. Garrison insists she must leave the hospital. The members of the staff have tried to calm her and convince her to change her mind. She has just been told that she has the sickle cell trait, and the doctors have advised her to have a hysterectomy. She already has three children and one is in the hospital now, being treated for a sickle-cell crisis. The child is very sick; Ms. Garrison is disturbed not only about the fact that she must give up her dream of having a large family, but also she is worried about her very sick child. She was admitted to the hospital for a D and C only, when several of the staff doctors began to urge her to have the hysterectomy.

Ms. Garrison is black.

SITUATION #5: Mrs. King has just had minor surgery and is anticipating her discharge from the hospital within a few days. She is not happy. On the contrary, she is making everyone's life miserable. She is demanding, leaning on her light from morning through half the night: her bed is too high, her bed is too low, where are her tissues, the television set isn't working properly, etc. She receives every effort to help her ungraciously, with hostile criticism about how long people take, how inefficient they are, etc.

Her manner with her doctor reveals tight-lipped enmity. She says almost nothing to him, but her attitude is clear. Once she was heard shouting to her husband that she had been forced into the hospital against her will and into surgery for no reason at all. She feels she had been made to suffer unnecessarily.

SITUATION #6: Because of persistent discomfort in her back and side, a woman has been admitted to the hospital for a diagnostic work-up. She is an attractive lady, tanned by the summer sun, bright-eyed and friendly. She says she doesn't feel ill enough to stay in bed, so each morning she washes, combs her hair, puts on lipstick and a bright yellow robe, and walks along the corridor, stopping to speak to patients and staff on the way. In the afternoons, she is too busy to leave her room. Since she is eighty years old and the head of a large family, friends and family members come in a continuing stream.

Discussion

The first and the sixth situations are substantially the same, despite the differences in the ages of the man and woman. Both have minor symptoms; both are pleasant, independent individuals. Both seem to be enjoying life, involved with the people around them.

Do you see a pattern in your observations about one patient that is quite different from the pattern of your observations about the other? Do you make different assumptions and come to different conclusions because one is younger than the other? Are there things you would like to know about one that you wouldn't care to know about the other? Why? Is it the age difference that matters? The sex difference? The different expectations about the course of the illness?

Actually, the young man underwent surgery, was found to have a malignant tumor of the kidney, and had the kidney removed. The cause of the old woman's discomfort was not discovered. She went home with a bottle of aspirin and eventually her symptoms disappeared.

In the second and fourth situations are people whose lives at this moment show some parallels. Both Ms. Milton and Ms. Garrison are very unhappy. Both have seriously handicapped children, whose troubles are genetically linked. Both have been hoping to have other children. Yet, they have been advised against this. In addition, Ms. Milton is afraid that she may have cancer. Ms. Milton's fear of surgery seems to have no parallel with Ms. Garrison until you learn that Ms. Garrison finally agreed to the hysterectomy. She died three days after surgery. Ms. Milton left the hospital without surgery.

What were your reactions to the situation of each patient? Were you quite sure that only one should have no more children, or quite sure that both should undergo the suggested surgery? Was your opinion influenced by the race of the patient? Did you think that one or the other might die? Was there any hint in your reactions that might be interpreted as different dying trajectories for these two women? What would the differences in your observations and comments have been if you had been able to foretell the endings to these two stories?

Both Mr. Lupton (Situation #3) and Mrs. King (Situation #5) left the hospital within a week. Though Mr. Lupton was, according to the nurses, on a speedy dying trajectory, he did not die during that admission nor during any of his three admissions in the ensuing year. Mrs. King was also readmitted to the hosiptal three times in the following year.

Both Mr. Lupton and Mrs. King were, during the time they were in contact with medical personnel, in very similar positions, demonstrating very similar behaviors. In what ways did the differences in their dying trajectories affect the pattern of your observations in these two situations?

Selective perception

When we encounter a person or a situation, we usually respond in terms of what we expect that person or situation to be like. In stereotypic thinking, we assume on the basis of irrelevant cues and learned errors that our expectations are accurate. Selective perception is closely associated with stereotypic thinking. We stereotype so easily because we are able to exclude from our awareness certain aspects of the person or situation that do not conform to our preconceptions. We forget those things that interfere with our expectations and distort others to make them fit. This kind of forgetting and exclusion is selective perception.

One example of selective perception was recently observed in a hospital. A woman was brought to the hospital and treated with great "enthusiasm." This treatment caused her to contract even more serious difficulties than the ones with which she was admitted. When her own physician arrived, he was given the reasons for the extreme treatment: the woman had been having respiration difficulty and she was dying. Another physician, who was visiting the patient in the next bed and who witnessed the treatment, told the doctor that she saw no indication at all of respiratory difficulty; the woman was certainly in pain, but her breathing under the circumstances was normal. Three other people who happened to be observing could see no evidence of breathing difficulty (though they were not physicians). One was a nurse, one an aide, one just another visitor.

The history of breathing difficulty remained on the patient's chart, and subsequent treatments were undertaken as if there were no question of its accuracy. The woman's own physician, though he had two sets of conflicting reports, continued to act as if he had only the first report. When members of the family (who had been told of the incident) kept reminding him that it was possible—perhaps probable—that the patient had had no respiratory difficulty at all, he did not acknowledge their opinion. When he finally sent his report to another city to which the patient was moved, he made a point to emphasize the "respiratory difficulty."

It appears that the attending physician never made a conscious decision to accept one version of the patient's condition over the other. It really did seem, after a short while, that he had completely forgotten the conflicting version.

If you would like to see for yourself how inaccurate perceptions can be, there is a short exercise you and your colleagues might try. Pick a room in the hospital where there is usually a great deal of activity: people coming and going, patients and staff dealing with each other in a variety of activities, white people, Black people, men, women. Six students should walk into the room and look around for two or three minutes trying to get a clear idea of who is in the room and what they are doing. Do not speak to each other or to anyone else.

At the end of three minutes, leave the room and go to a place where you can record your observation. Each of you, without any discussion, should write down everything you remember about the room, its occupants, and their behavior.

When you have finished, compare your accounts. You will probably find many things you observed that others did not, and vice versa. It is also likely that you thought some things were very significant, while you thought others unimportant. An incident that someone else describes you may have seen completely differently.

No one lied, or set out to deceive. It is just that you brought to your observation different experiences and expectations. What really happened was filtered through these individual differences.

Another way of becoming aware of this process of selective perception is described in two of my other books (*Effective Interaction in Contemporary Nursing,* Prentice-Hall; *Intergroup Relations for the Classroom Teacher,* Intext). A variation of that one is to have only one person go into the room full of activity. After two or three minutes he should return to the group and ask four people to leave the room. She should then tell the group what she observed. They should make no comments or ask any questions; they should merely listen. One of them calls a person from outside and tells him what she heard. The third person tells the fourth person; the fourth tells the fifth; and the fifth tells the sixth. As the rest of the group listens to the telling and re-telling, they should note how the story changes. At the end, they can discuss the changes, again bearing in mind that nobody lied—and that *everybody* distorted.

Given heightened awareness of human susceptibility to this kind of distortion, and given also increased insight into the nature of one's own distortions, error in perception may be substantially reduced. However, one needs to mantain eternal vigilance.

Prejudice

Here is another example of the way selective perception can affect a dying trajectory. In this situation, a man died in a way he neither wanted nor needed to die, as a result of a staff's prejudice that caused them to perceive a situation inaccurately.

Mr. Madison was brought to the hospital in a police ambulance. He had been found convulsing on a city street. The neighborhood where he was found was one of very poor Black people. Mr. Madison was a young Black man. Although someone had apparently called the police when they saw him thrashing about on the ground, most of the bystand-

ers would not come close to him. When the police arrived, the seizure
was almost over. The police first assumed that he had been in a fight
and spent some time trying to find out what had happened from the
people nearby. They got vague reports that "He was just layin' there,
makin' noises." To more insistent questions, they shrugged. No one knew
how he got there.

The police finally took him to the hospital, announcing in the emergency room that he was probably full of some rotten dope. *"They* buy
anything; who knows what the stuff is half the time?"

The hospital staff worked quickly to save his life. Once he opened his
eyes to protest feebly that he was "sick . . . very sick." One doctor responded: "You're sick, all right. You may never come out of this. What
did you take? Tell us what you took."

"Nothing," he said. "I'm just sick."

"Well, if you won't tell us what you took, we won't be able to save
you. You'll die. Do you understand what I'm saying? You'll die."

"I'm just sick. I'm just sick," the young man continued to protest.

Mr. Madison died of a stroke with massive brain damage, without the
comfort of having his family with him or of having medical practitioners
that were inclined to comfort him. Their "treatment" probably hastened
his death. Their assumption that because of his age, his race, and his
neighborhood he must have been drugged, prevented them from assigning
him a more realistic trajectory.

Behavioral consequences of a defined trajectory: a case study

Recently, the author had occasion to witness what appeared to be an
entire hospital's attitude toward a group of patients whose dying trajectory was perceived inaccurately. The distorted perception was apparently a function of cultural bias that had been reinforced by the
unique hospital situation, and resulted in behavior that was so inappropriate as to become destructive.

This hospital is a new, heavily-endowed facility, equipped with the
most modern diagnostic and treatment facilities, and staffed with a full
complement of health personnel on every level of preparation. Its one-
and two-bed rooms are beautifully furnished with every convenience for
the comfort and care of patients. The hospital's intensive care unit boasts
a separate section for special care for patients who need round-the-clock
treatment and observation, but who have some chance of recovery. The

rest of the intensive care section is for people who need even more of such special care, but who are also expected to recover.

A team of prestige nurses rules this unit with an iron—and rather nasty —hand, reiterating the unit's rules to families, inhalation therapists, technicians, aides, and attendants with a consistent and overbearing hostility that does not seem to lessen even when they approach their patients. Other nurses in the hospital resent the attitude of this team, characterizing it as consisting of "recent graduates who think no one knows anything about nursing except them."

The hostile attitude of the nurses in intensive care has been assumed by the other personnel in the unit; however, their hostility is directed only against the patient's families, and takes the form of refusing to respond to questions (even when the questions refer to information about visiting hours), brusquely ordering people to "line up," "keep away from the door," and talking about "those people" to their fellow workers in full view of the targets of their contempt.

When it is decided that a patient will not recover, he is moved across the hall to another section, where his family may see him during regular visiting hours instead of intensive-care hours: five minutes every hour *on the hour,* for only one visitor. Although the staff has decided that it is no longer any use to give this patient more than minimal care, his family is still often instructed not to let the patient know he is dying. The result is a ghastly ludicrous game played by dying patients and their families consisting of guessing who knows what and pretending the truth is not known. The game is played with red eyes, much surreptitious blowing of noses, and frequent precipitous dashes out of the room. Volunteers, who are so ubiquitous at this hospital that they seem to make up fifty percent of the staff, keep reassuring everyone that "they're doing everything they can," and exhorting people to "calm down," and "don't let the patient see you crying."

One man, so ill that he would have had to be comatose not to recognize his desperate state, was the center of this idiocy for several days. He said little or nothing, seeming to focus all his waning energy on drawing each painful breath. During a lull in the activity, when he and the patient in the next bed were alone for a moment, he said to me between gasps for breath, "It's good to close your eyes and sleep forever. I wish I could do that." Outside the room, the man's son was crying as he kept reassuring his mother that "Dad will come out of this; he's strong." The patient's wife was crying in bursts of terror, confiding to every stranger who would listen that she just knew it was something terrible, but that no one would tell her the truth. The daughter-in-law furiously berated the woman for being selfish ("Dad will see you crying") and for making a spectacle of herself in public. While this was going on, the patient wished only for the peace of endless sleep.

In other parts of the hospital, the day to day business of hospital care went on just as efficiently, with a curious difference. The difference was that sixty-six percent of the patients were expected to become severely ill or to die within a relatively short period of time. (This was a large general hospital set in the heart of a small city.)

The background of this perception of the dying trajectories of so many of the patients lies in the nature of the patient population: about two-thirds of the population was over sixty-five years of age. This characteristic of the population was a natural result of the city's population, which is made up of a majority of old people. Most of them live on a fixed income from the social security program; others supplement their income with small pensions or assistance from their families. Some very few take part-time jobs that are not beyond their limited physical abilities.

It is an old-people's city, and the younger people who must interact with the old people do so in terms of the general society's perception of the aged. Although the city provides reduced-fare privileges for the old, bus drivers are impatient and grossly impolite, and are not above slamming a bus door on an old man who is moving too slowly, or starting the bus with a violent jerk because on old woman peering around for a seat does not immediately respond to the shouted order to "sit down, lady!" Storekeepers and clerks, who are usually willing to listen to complaints and answer endless questions by people of their own age, almost literally throw purchases at old people, will answer no questions about price or quality of foods and other products, and become hostile at any suggestion of complaint.

Landlords in the city, most of whom own and run small residential hotels with cooking facilities, engage in outright thievery and rely on the powerlessness of their tenants to escape apprehension by the legal authorities. They may contract for a monthly rent that includes supplying towels and having a maid change the bed linens once a week. However, they will not hesitate to cut off such services—and the hot water as well. When the tenants protest, they are told they are free to move if they do not like the situation. Since moving means they must forfeit the month's rent they have paid as a security bond, they live out the contract year in discomfort and sometimes anguish. It is not unusual for them to carry their few belongings from hotel to hotel, year after year, hoping that this year they will find an honest landlord.

Even youngsters, going to and from school on buses, on bicycles, and on foot, show an ugly contempt for the old people they pass and jostle. One cross look or word of complaint will bring down on the old man or woman a volley of obscene verbal abuse or a giggling attack of juvenile sarcasm taken up first by one child, then by another, until everyone in the crowd has had a turn.

This, then, is the ambience of the city from which are drawn both patients and staff. And this general pattern of interaction between the old and the young seems directly related to the way the hospital staff views its patients. There is an off-hand casualness in the perception of patients that, curiously enough, stops short of the actual medical treatment. That is, the expectation that patiens have not long to live no matter what is done for them, does not prevent physicians and nurses from diligently applying the latest knowledge, skill, and machinery in their medical and surgical treatment. The errors were made outside of the actual medical procedures, errors that were a function of the generalized dying trajectory defined by the staff.

For example, an eighty-year-old man was brought into the hospital by ambulance. He had apparently suffered a seizure of unknown etiology. He had almost complete aphasia. His communication was unintelligible, although the affect of the sounds he made seemed to be related to what he was trying to say. He spoke and seemed very perplexed and disturbed when people did not understand what he said. It was difficult to tell if he could understand what people said to him. He followed directions sporadically, and then he did so with movements that only approximated what he was told to do.

The attitude of the hospital toward him and his condition might be characterized by a vast, institutional shrug of the shoulders. After all, he *was* eighty years old. When family members insisted that, until he had been found in this condition, he was perfectly all right in every way, the response was generally one of polite skepticism. After a series of routine tests, it was announced that he had massive brain damage, diabetes, Parkinson's disease, and that he was paralyzed on the left side, with no ability to use his left arm and leg. "Obviously," a physician told the man's daughter, "you will have to put him into an institution that offers custodial care. It will be like caring for a baby, and you would not want to do that."

Members of the man's family protested that he had seen a doctor regularly and had no indication of diabetes. The doctor shrugged his shoulders. The daughter said that five minutes before the diagnosis of paralysis the patient had moved his arm and leg with no apparent difficulty. The doctor might never have heard. The patient got out of bed and headed for the bathroom, his stride hesistant but normal, no different from what it had been for thirty years. The neurologist smiled as he passed and repeated, "He has Parkinson's."

Two days after his admission, he had another seizure. His daughter was at his bedside. A nurse poked her head in the door, saw what was happening and said, "I'll get someone." She wandered away, never to be seen again. An hour later a physician appeared and made notes on the patient's chart, apparently based on what the nurse had seen from the door.

Two weeks later, the patient was taken home. He had *none* of the illnesses or debilities diagnosed; the cause of the seizure was still unknown; he spoke perfectly well. Though his memory of recent events was impaired, he was apparently improving. The medical staff was literally open-mouthed with surprise. One doctor who left on a holiday for several days said he couldn't believe his eyes when he got back. When pressed about his diagnoses of diabetes and paralysis, he suddenly heard them paging him.

Despite the mistakes, this was a good hospital, with a well-trained nursing staff, and physicians who had reputations for considerable skill and knowledge. The obviously bad medicine practiced was simply a function of the city's attitude toward old people: 1) They are expected to have a variety of ills. 2) Four-score years is a reasonably sufficient length of time to have lived. 3) Old people who linger beyond their expected span need to be put away.

Lest you think this case has been singled out and is only an isolated instance in the way trajectories are perceived in this hospital, here are records of conversatons with staff members that give additional clues to the prevailing attitudes:

Interview #1

INTERVIEWER: You work almost entirely with old people. Do you like this kind of patient population?

NURSE: Well, actually, I majored in peds. I was sure I'd spend my professional life working with children. I really loved it.

INTERVIEWER: Didn't you find it difficult to make the change? From one extreme to the other?

NURSE: Oh, no. There's really no difference. I get along just fine with old people. The psychology is the same—for children and for old people.

INTERVIEWER: The same? Surely a man who has worked for 60 years, reared a family and experienced a full life does not have the thoughts and feelings of a child?

NURSE: (smiling sweetly and pointing to a patient in the violent throes of a senile psychosis) I get along just fine with him. I know how to make him listen and do as I say.

On the surface, it would appear that perceiving old people as children negates the proposition that the staff stereotypes its patients in dying trajectories. However, this may merely be an aspect of a curious analogy made by at least one researcher in the field (Kübler-Ross). She likens the peaceful end of life, with the need for increasing sleep and the lack of concern with the world, to the beginning of life and the infant's similar need for sleep and lack of worldly involvement. Perhaps—unconsciously —this nurse, and others like her, see the aged as children in terms of this same analogy. If this is true, then the way they define the old person's dying trajectory follows logically: the only appropriate trajectory is a speedy one.

Interview #2

INTERVIEWER: I notice you have a large room for physical therapy, but there are very few patients using it.

THERAPIST: They're not very rehabilitation-minded here. It's more just treat them and send them home to sit.

INTERVIEWER: You mean they don't believe in physical therapy?

THERAPIST: Oh, they believe in it for younger people. It's just for old people they don't think anyone wants to be bothered. The patients resist a lot—they have trouble changing the way they walk and things like that. Their families don't have the time to do exercises with them—and they don't have the time to keep bringing them here.

INTERVIEWER: It sounds almost as if you're saying that old people are going to die soon, anyway, that it all hardly seems worth the trouble.

THERAPIST: Oh, that's not it, I'm sure. Nobody wants anyone to die. But I must admit that there are patients whose physical deterioration could be slowed down with regular therapy. Even mentally they'd be better off. They get so discouraged when their movement is severely limited. They can't do anything for themselves.

Interview #3

ORTHOPEDIST: The X-ray shows the head of the thigh has pushed into the pelvis and fractured it.

PATIENT: Will it heal up all right?

ORTHOPEDIST: Well, we could operate. How old are you—eighty? You don't want to bother with surgery. You'll just have to live with it.

SISTER OF PATIENT: He's in good health, otherwise, isn't he?

ORTHOPEDIST: Sure, sure. If he has pain, let him take the pills.

PATIENT: Will I be able to walk all right?

ORTHOPEDIST: How much walking do you have to do? Where do you
    want to walk? Don't put any weight on that leg.

(Orthopedist approached by technician. He leaves, discussing the technician's problem, leaving the patient and his sister to wander out of the
office.)

What was communicated to the observer was another example of a
dying trajectory that reflected an attitude toward old people. There was
no serious consideration or discussion by the orthopedist of the patient's
suitability for corrective surgery. The implicaton was clear that, at the
age of eighty, the appropriate trajectory was a speedy one, and the only
reasonable expectation was that the patient would sit and wait for the
end of that trajectory.

An article in the New York Times (6/23/74) points out that "the
most persistent efforts to legalize euthanasia take place in Florida, [a
state that has] a disproportionate number of old people [in its population.]" Other researches indicate that the pressures for "freedom to die
with dignity" are being applied by relatively young people, not by those
who by virtue of their advanced age are nearer to dying. It is not inconceivable that the rejection and neglect of old people in our society
and our concern with overpopulation may result in public decision-
making about the "appropriate" time for an individual to die. The implications are terrifying.

Isolating the attitudes related to defining trajectories

Below are some brief descriptions of circumstances that require a defini-
tion or evaluation of the dying trajectory. It is suggested that you respond
to these circumstances by yourself, without discussing your ideas with
anyone else. Also write down the feelings, thoughts, and ideas that occur
to you, so that you will have a record of your responses for a systematic
evaluation. When you have finished writing, you may read the discussion
that follows.

1. A patient is brought into a hospital severely hurt from an automobile
   accident. Quickly list the questions that pop into your mind that you
   want to ask about him.

2. A patient's only chance of relief from a fatal heart disease is a new and complicated surgical procedure requiring the cooperative efforts of top cardiac surgeons. What do you need to know about the patient before you can decide in your own mind whether or not he should have the surgery?

3. A patient is scheduled for surgery, but he is given only a small chance of surviving. How do you justify in your own mind that this particular patient should be encouraged to take the risk of the surgery?

4. A patient is being kept alive by a respirator. What would you want to know about him before you could make a decision to discontinue such "heroic" measures?

5. At what age should a person be permitted to die if he wants to?

6. A patient who is eighty years old has been brought to the hospital with a broken hip. He is in great pain, but he is apparently in complete control of his faculties. He insists on medication to control the pain so that he may "go to sleep forever." He refuses to permit any other treatment. How hard would you try to convince him to permit treatment? List the arguments you would use.

7. A well-known public figure commits suicide. It is learned that he had just been diagnosed as suffering from cancer. List the feelings you have when you learn about his suicide.

8. If no doctor were present for miles and you had a patient who seemed to have suddenly died, under what circumstances would you feel free to conclude that he was dead and thus to discontinue emergency aid? Include in your answer information other than that dealing with the person's physical condition.

9. If there were a sudden failure in the equipment that is keeping a patient alive, what would you have to know about the patient before you engaged in heroic attempts to provide other means for prolonging his life? (Such heroic attempts might involve convincing other staff members—such as physicians—that they must do something.)

Discussion

Check back through your responses and see if you can identify a pattern. For example, is the age of the patient always an important consideration for you? Why? Do you feel it is more important to prolong the trajectory of a young person than an old person? What is the cut-off point for you? There are many physicians who consider sixty-five the reasonable age for discontinuing productivity. Is this your view, also? On what do you base this view—what society demands, or what people over sixty-five have been able to demonstrate they can do?

Does your judgment of a dying trajectory ever involve the past accomplishments of a patient? The social value of the patient to the community? The wealth of the patient? If yes, does this mean that medical personnel are in a position to make life and death decisions based on their perception of how important a person is? What, then, of those medical people who were taught to value people according to how much money they had, or to reject people because of their race or religion? What about the doctor who detests alcoholics because his mother was one? What about the nurse who thinks drug addicts are weak, and so contemptible?

Does it matter to you whether or not the patient has a family? Why? Does the dying trajectory ever depend on the size of the patient's family? The presence of the patient's family? The forcefulness or self-assertion of the patient's family? Why should the patient's family be a significant factor in the dying trajectory?

After examining your own attitudes, you may wish to discuss some of the questions with other members of your group. Form groups of eight or nine people, so that everyone has an opportunity to speak, and feels relatively comfortable in expressing his feelings.

If, in your discussion, you begin to recognize significant differences between your own attitudes and those of people in the wider society, you might, as a group, consider making a commitment to resist the effects of attitudes you reject. There is more chance of effecting change if likeminded individuals work together, giving each other support and strength.

Clarifying values related to defining trajectories

Below are several points of view related to defining dying trajectories. Pick the point of view that most nearly approximates your own. You may change or refine it in any way, until you are able to say, "This is where I stand."

1. The patient really has no contribution to make in defining his own dying trajectory. He simply does not have the necessary scientific information, and so must depend on those who do have this information to define his trajectory.
2. The value of the patient to society at large and to the community must figure prominently in the decisions made about treatment, comfort-care, and nature of the facilities provided for the patient. Even hospital rules must be applied flexibly to reflect the social status of the patient.
3. It is only natural that the life of a young person be more highly valued

than the life of an old person. Consequently, the dying trajectory—the time and the nature of the patient's course to death—will be affected by his age.

4. The value of the patient *to himself* must figure significantly in the decisions that will affect the course of his dying. Only if he is comatose should medical personnel rely on those who know him best to gain information concerning his feelings about living and dying. However, secondhand information may be misleading because people may be influenced by their own feelings and needs in their perceptions of even those very close to them.

Discussion

You need not share your values with the other people in your group immediately, if you would like to take more time to consider just where you do stand on this issue. The point of the above exercise is to clarify your own values, to sort out your own points of view. As you think about the various aspects of the issue, it might help you to make a choice if you consider the consequences—in individual cases and to our society—of each point of view.

Eventually, you should begin to talk to your colleagues about your choice. Values are not really functional until we are ready to take a public stand on them.

section four

Death at
Different Ages

chapter nine

———◄•►———

Treating
the Dying Child

Attitudes

Sometimes, attitudes toward death and the dying become somewhat
blurred, and it is difficult to determine the rationality of certain behaviors.
For example, most of us are very disturbed when we meet young people
who are dying. When patients are older, we face the fact of their imminent death with somewhat more equanimity. Superficially, this kind of
differentiated behavior might seem to make good sense. If we view life
realistically, we know that our time on earth is limited and the older we
get the sooner we will die. We say of a seventy-year-old man, "He has
lived his life." The implication is that it is time for him to die.

However, we must look closely at the behavioral consequences of such
an attitude. Is it possible that we are less accepting of the anger and grief
of a sixty-year-old woman faced with her own death than we are with similar emotions in a twenty-five-year-old woman? We feel a responsive pang
when a thirty-year-old man exclaims, "Why me?" Do we feel the same
emotion when a sixty-five-year-old man cries, "No! It's not happening to
me!"? Would we be willing to take as much time and trouble to help an
old man die as we are to help a young man die?

Conversely, is there something about our feeling of "tragedy" and great
sorrow when a young person dies that might make us avoid a young dying
person, and find it easier to work with an older person who is dying?

Is the anguish we feel when we encounter a dying child so great that we completely forget the feelings and perceptions of the child as we respond to his dying by overwhelming him with gifts and pampering and arch cheerfulness?

It may be significant that a survey of physicians' attitudes (Scott, *Medical Opinion,* May, 1974) reveals that almost one-third of the pediatricians questioned said they hadn't really thought about their own deaths. No other physician-specialist group questioned had such a large percentage respond in this way. One can only guess the personal problems faced by these physicians when they must diagnose imminent death for a small patient. Although the researcher who made this finding called the pediatricians' attitude "mortal optimism," the attitude reveals more of fear and denial than it does of hope and joy connoted by the word optimism. One must conclude that the adult who has managed to avoid thinking about his own death will have great difficulty accepting the inevitability of a child's death. Certainly the openness and acceptance recommended by other workers with children is likely to be resisted.

People such as Kavanaugh insist that "Knowledge is kindness, ignorance is cruel." Children learn very quickly that they are dying, from the signs around them or even from playmates who hear their parents talk. The hollow cheerfulness and pampering of adults merely isolates them and makes them feel guilty for that unknown evil that is causing their punishment. The dying child has a right to be included in the feelings and anxieties that the people around him are experiencing. It is not fair to force him to grieve alone because adults are not prepared to accept his awareness and his grief.

By the time a child is seven years old, he probably suspects that he himself will die one day. As early as the age of four he may already have some partial notion that death is associated with sadness. The misconception that many adults harbor is that children never think of death and that they know nothing about it; however, the evidence we have does not support this opinion. Children know about death, are interested in it, and have feelings of sadness and fear at evidences of death in their lives.

Such evidences are all around them. They see death on television and in the movies. They hear discussion of death in the news. Even their nursery rhymes and fairy tales deal with death in both fanciful and realistic ways. Some evidences of death are more personal and direct, as when an animal or an insect dies, or when a playmate disappears or a family member is mourned. Younger children are often confused into believing that the departure is only temporary, and they voice repeatedly their expectations that the dead person will come back. This confusion is based partly on the fact that they are overgeneralizing from their personal experiences: people do go away and come back again; playmates hide and are discovered with glee in games of hide-and-seek. However, this error in generalization is compounded and reinforced by the fears and circumlocutions of adults. When the child is told that Grandma has gone away, or that his small brother was taken to heaven by God, the implication is clear: the missing person is on a trip; there is no reason to suppose that the loved one will not return one day.

It is possible that children, early in their lives, can learn to deal with death more realistically than previous generations. Unfortunately, the topic of death is usually surrounded with more taboos in the school and home than are the subjects of sex and race relations. Adults make it clear that these topics are not to be mentioned, and insist that children have no interest in them.

The sad fact is that when a child is dying, we can no longer afford to delude ourselves. The child has known about death; he probably has guessed by now that he is dying. What can we do to prevent his isolation and make him less fearful and more accepting of his dying?

Exercises in Listening

1. Accurate reflection

There is some evidence that, unless an adult takes the initiative in discussing the subject, a child will maintain the fiction that he does not think about death. In addition, those who have worked with dying children remind us often that we must listen carefully to a dying child if we are to detect the subtle cues about death that creep into his words and behavior in spite of his wariness. Thus, if we are to be helpful to the dying child, it would seem necessary to develop skills in listening and in encouraging openness and freedom to express feelings.

Following is an exercise in listening that most people find so difficult and frustrating that it is clear what our great problem in listening is: we simply are more concerned with what *we* have to say than with what anyone else is saying! Therefore, we are usually uncertain about what people are trying to tell us.

In a group of about eight people, sit in a circle and discuss a topic of general interest. Perhaps you should not choose an emotional subject, since you are trying to learn a new skill and this might interfere with the discussion. If you have very strong feelings about the topic you will need to get them out without the artificiality of being limited by the rules of the game. You might wish to choose one of the following questions, taken from a Problem Census done with a group of experienced nurses:

How do you get an old person who doesn't want to live to take a hand in his own recovery?

I've noticed that most people are very uncomfortable when they have to talk to a patient who is dying. How professional is *that?*

How do you help a young woman who thinks her life is over because she had a leg amputated?

What do you say to a patient who says he wants to die? *

Have your discussion just as you would any other discussion, with one exception: you may not say anything until you have accurately reflected what the previous speaker has said. When you want to speak, you should turn to the previous speaker and say: "Did you mean to say . . . ?" Fill in the blank with what you thought you heard her say. She may nod, to indicate that you understand her, in which case you may go on with your own contribution to the discussion. If she says, "No," you may try again, "Did you mean to say . . . ?" If she says, "No," again, someone else may try. The previous speaker *must not repeat what she has said.* If no one can accurately reflect what she has said, then she may try to say it again. The group can decide if the problem was that they were not listening well, or that the speaker was not really saying what she thought she was. However, it is better not to spend too long on this, because it is often impossible to determine whose perceptions were accurate and whose were not.

Sometimes we are not skillful in letting others know what is on our minds. Consequently, when we think we are saying one thing, we are really saying something quite different. This accounts for at least some of the errors made in reflecting back.

One way to establish clear communication is to check with the speaker in any conversation to see if you understand him before you rush to make your own contribution. Reflecting back to him what you think he has said will give him a chance to correct and clarify, so that when you finally do make your comments, they are truly responsive. You will then be able to (1) use what he has said as a basis to extend the thought or idea, so that a new perspective enters the shared communication; (2) give him a straightforward answer to a question he is asking; (3) express appreciation for a feeling he is revealing; or (4) remain silent and listen because that seems to be the needed response. None of this is possible unless you know what the speaker is trying to say.

When you have had several opportunities to practice accurate reflection, perhaps your group might like to discuss the following situation.

* Charlotte Epstein, *Effective Interaction in Contemporary Nursing* (Englewood Cliffs, N.J.: Prentice-Hall, Inc., 1974).

Though you are not, at this time, constrained to reflect back before each time you want to speak, you should make sure that you do know what people are really saying before you jump in to argue, advise, or even agree. In the course of the discussion, if you feel that you are not accurately perceiving what someone is trying to say, let him try to clarify his point before you respond.

> Joyce is eleven years old. She has cancer in the lungs. Her mother keeps telling her that when her cough clears up she will come home.
> As they work each shift, the nurses continually tell Joyce that she is looking better. They tell each other the same thing. There is never any suggestion in their conversations about Joyce that she is dying. Their exchange deals mostly with transmitting the notes about her medication and physical care.
> Most of the interaction between the child and the nurses is limited to a few necessary words of direction and admonition. They also speak little to Joyce's mother. They never talk about the illness if they can help it. They are kind, but they maintain a certain "professional" distance between themselves and Joyce and her mother.
> The nurses tend to Joyce's physical needs before and after visiting hours. When Joyce's mother is there, they are usually busy with paper work in the small office behind the nurse's station.
> It is interesting to note that, although nothing is said, everyone who comes to work first looks in on Joyce—as if they are checking to see if she is still there. They do not smile with relief or say anything when they see her; they just go on about their business, sometimes with a barely perceptible tightening around the mouth.
> How do you feel about this situation?

2. Eye contact

Checking the accuracy of your perception of what a person is saying is a way of encouraging that person to continue his communication with you. It gives him evidence that you are really listening to him and trying to understand him. Here is another exercise to help you practice behavior that makes it clear that you are listening to what the other person is saying. Divide your group in half and separate the two halves. Each person in one of the two groups should think of a great loss that he has experienced at some time in his life—a relative, a friend, a lover, a possession. Spend a few moments reliving the experience; try to recall the feelings associated with that loss.

Each person should pick one person from the other half of the group that he thinks he can trust with his experience. He should tell this person about his loss in some detail—how he felt about it, how he still feels. *Do not read beyond this line until you have completed the exercise.*

This direction is for the listeners only—for those persons chosen to hear about the losses of the other half of the group. While you are listening to this person who is telling you about his loss, *avoid looking at him.* Do not make eye contact. You may turn your head away, look over his shoulder, examine your fingernails—look anywhere except at his face until he has finished talking.

When each person has told his story, the group should reconvene. The people who expressed their losses should respond to the following questions:

1. How did you feel while you were telling your story?
2. How interested do you think your partner was in what you were saying?
3. Were you able to tell the whole story? Why or why not?
4. If you left out part of the story, can you explain the significance of leaving out that particular part?
5. You picked your partner originally because you trusted him; how do you feel about him now?

You might wish to exchange stories now with a member of your half of the group, since your whole group has been subjected to the inattention of the other group. While this is going on, the first group of listeners should summarize the effects of not looking at the speaker. It might be helpful to write this summary with a felt pen on large sheets of newsprint and tape it to the wall for the duration of your seminar as a reminder of what you have observed.

When all the storytellers have finished, they may examine the summary and make any additions they feel are important in the light of the experience they have just had in telling their stories to listeners who *do* pay attention.

3. Other evidences of listening

To take your discussion a step further, see if you can identify some other listener behaviors that help to assure the speaker that he is being listened to. What did the speakers see and hear that made them feel comfortable—or uncomfortable? What do you think of the following behaviors?

1. The listener nods his head as if he hears something that is making a particular impression on him.
2. The listener says, "I can imagine how you felt."
3. The listener murmurs, "How terrible!"

4. The listener puts his hand to his head, as if he feels, for a moment, the pain of the teller.
5. The listener leans back, away from the teller.
6. The listener moves closer to the teller.
7. The listener looks very tense and uncomfortable.
8. The listener asks many questions, ostensibly to keep the speaker focused on what is important in the story.
9. The listener tells about an experience he had that was very similar to the speaker's experience. (Does the time of this behavior make a difference in the effect it has? That is, if the listener tells his story as soon as the speaker has completed the details of his story, would it make the speaker feel differently than if the speaker has had some time to repeat some of the details and to express again some of his feelings? In other words, does the speaker have time to repeat some elements of his story, or is he immediately forced to listen to the other person?)
10. The listener touches the teller.

Encouraging communication

Because this section concerns communicating with children, we should use techniques that children are more likely to respond to than adults. Sometimes, such techniques require the preparation of materials that are not generally associated with nursing. It may at first seem inappropriate behavior for a nurse until one realizes that, ideally, both teaching and nursing are helping professions. The truly effective teacher refrains from "covering" material or disseminating bits of information. Instead, she encourages the student to become involved in knowing himself and others, and in developing skills for living in a way that is satisfying. Similarly, the effective nurse helps the patient to become involved in making his life as satisfying and productive as possible even though the patient is ill.

1. Comic strips

If your small patient can write, you can give him an opportunity to reveal what is on his mind that he is almost sure to take advantage of. (As a matter of fact, you might enjoy this activity yourself.) By putting his *own* words in the mouths of comic characters, the child not only reveals his feelings, but also may dissociate himself from those feelings. For example, any time your patient wishes to retract something he regrets revealing, he may easily do so: "*I* don't feel this way; Krazy Kat is the one who kicked his mother!" Thus, the completed strips may afford clues for further questioning or for discussing subjects on the child's mind.

To begin this exercise, cut out several comic strips in the newspaper. Take each strip and cut out and discard the conversation in the balloons. Paste each strip on a piece of unlined paper. (Unused newsprint or wrapping paper will do.) Now you have characters into whose mouths you can put any words you wish and whose bodily stances you can interpret in any way you like.

If you want to test out this activity with your own group, have each person prepare one or two strips and then redistribute them so that the original words of the strip are not so familiar to the people working on them. Each person should have the comic strip characters deal with a subject that relates to your seminar on dying. Or you may decide to fill in the balloons with any words that relate to what is on your mind or to something that bugs you.

When everyone is finished, collect the strips and shuffle them so that the authors cannot be identified. The group should select and study one strip at a time to develop a plan for helping the author of the strip 1) express himself further on the subject of his comic strip, 2) answer his questions, 3) feel better about himself as a person.

In order to develop a plan that fulfills these three objectives, follow these steps:

1. Identify the topic of concern and the situational details that relate to the topic.
2. Identify the cues that reveal feelings about the topic and define those feelings as they are revealed in the strip.
3. Identify the cues that reveal the feelings that the author has about himself and define those feelings as they are revealed in the strip.
4. Formula the author's questions—those that are implicit as well as those that are explicit.

In addition, develop strategies and materials for helping each other utilize what has been learned about encouraging, listening, and responding.

Once you have developed plans to help the several authors of the comic strips, you might like to test them. One person who *thinks* he understands an author's feelings should pretend to be that author. Another person who wishes to test the plan should play the role of the helping person who has the above three objectives. The rest of the group should observe the interaction between the two and take notes in three columns:

additional information and feelings revealed	evidences of satisfaction at having questions answered	evidences of increased acceptance of self

When the helping person decides he has completed the plan, the notes taken by the group should make it clear whether or not the objectives of the plan have been fulfilled. After sharing the results of your observations, you may decide to adjust your plan somewhat. Do not hesitate to do this. The objective of these exercises is to provide opportunities for learning skills, testing out what you have learned, and refining, so that when you are on the job the margin for errors of judgment and application is substantially reduced.

Below is an example of a comic strip and how it can be used. It was completed by a ten-year-old with leukemia. One day, the comic strip and a pencil were left on her bed tray with her usual books and toys. She picked up the comic strip without prompting and, after some thought, wrote in the balloons.

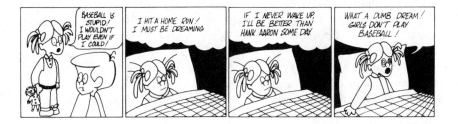

A nurse and I told her we were interested in what she had written and asked if we could borrow the strip. Following is our analysis of the content of the material. We did not attempt a profound symbolic analysis; we merely looked at her words for their explicit meaning and the feelings they seemed to reveal.

The child is concerned about her enforced lack of activity, her inability to play ball. Although, awake, she denies that she cares to play, she permits herself to dream of being a champion player.

Also on her mind is some thought of dying: "If I never wake up . . ." But she juxtaposes to this concern about dying, an advantage to be gained by never waking up: "I'll be better than Hank Aaron . . ."

She does not feel very good about herself: what she enjoys doing she *feels* is not for girls; what she likes to do is "stupid"; her dreams are "dumb."

At least two questions she seems to be asking are:

> Will I ever be able to play again?
> Am I going to die?

The plan was to give her an opportunity to talk about her past sports activities—playing baseball, ice skating—and the recognition and commendations she had received for skill in both activities. She was questioned about her exploits and her listeners shared with her the pleasure of her memories. They often expressed their appreciation of her sports ability, brought her newspaper clippings of sports events they thought would interest her, and directed her attention to television sports programs that she enjoyed watching. When two boys in the hospital unit had an argument about baseball, she was introduced to them as an expert—and she triumphed by settling the argument with some information she had and the boys did not.

In the discussion concerning her experiences, the plan noted that listeners should be alert for any overt expression of her concern about ever engaging in sports again. Finally, one day, she blurted: "I'll never be able to play baseball again, will I—or do any of those things?" Since the listeners had prepared themselves to expect this question, they did not succumb to the temptation to avoid answering or to lie. Their answer was that although the medicine she was taking made her feel reasonably comfortable, it could not make her so well that she could be very active.

The plan also noted that visitors should listen for cues that she was ready to discuss her feelings about dying. Thus, one day, when she said, "Sleeping is not so bad," the nurse was able to answer, "Tell me about sleeping." The child asked, "Is it like dying?"

Again, the nurse was prepared to stay with the patient. During the ensuing weeks, the child spoke more and more freely about dying. No one ever actually told her she was going to die, but she was obviously coming to terms with her condition as she talked out her feelings, asked for and received information, and had a hand to hold when she needed it.

The following comic strip was completed by a fourteen-year-old dying of cancer. Why don't *you* analyze it and then develop a plan for helping the patient? You may work alone if you prefer, although it is probably more realistic to work with a group, since a patient is rarely exposed to only one staff member, and everyone who comes into contact with him should be cognizant of the plan to help him. Also, sometimes an indi-

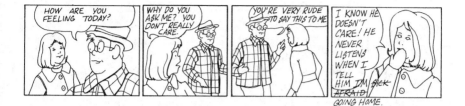

vidual cannot perceive every significant fact of a situation. Pooling the perceptions of a number of people helps clarify all aspects.

2. *Playing with dolls*

Every pediatrics unit has dolls, and most have "families" of small dolls that can be moved about easily. If a nurse puts the "family" out on a table and sits at the table with her patient playing with him, she is likely to hear and see evidences of how the child feels—about himself, his sisters and brothers, his parents, his stay in the hospital, other medical peronnel, and even the nurse herself.

One student nurse tried this with a six-year-old boy who recently had a leg amputated because of bone cancer and had just been admitted to the hospital again with evidence of metastases. She handed him the boy doll; he clutched it in one hand, looked up at her and said almost defiantly, "It's all right for boys to play with dolls!"

"Families have fathers and brothers," the student responded matter-of-factly, "just as they have mothers and sisters."

"I'm a brother," he said.

"Is that you?" she said, pointing to the doll in his hand.

He considered this for a moment, rolling the doll back and forth in his fingers. Then he said, "No. Two legs."

The student nurse felt she had inadvertently made an error in her plan with this patient: she thought she should have included a boy doll with one leg, so the child could identify with it. However, because the child was compelled to use the dolls that were there, he was able to reveal his feelings and ideas in the process of manipulating that character. There was no evidence that he had any great difficulty in identifying with the "family" just because the boy doll had two legs.

Over a period of fifteen minutes, he "made" the boy doll die; he had the mother crying (although in reality this child's mother repeatedly told

him he would be all right), he had all the other children lose arms,
legs, and other parts of their bodies. At the end of the session, he made
the student put out both her hands, palms up, and carefully laid the
"dead" doll in her hands and closed them softly and carefully over the
doll. Then he announced, "It's time to have some juice," and he asked
to be taken back to his bed.

For the rest of the day, he seemed content with the other children and
the TV. He was happy to see his mother when she came in, yet his attention focused on a game she had brought him. The next day, he
asked the student if they could play with the dolls again. He was ready
to continue his attempts to communicate with the person who had made
it clear that she was willing to try with him.

chapter ten

Treating the Patient Dying in the Prime of Life

Identifying with the patient

The patient who learns he is dying just when his life's ambitions are beginning to be realized touches most of us in a special way. After the uncertainties of adolescence, the agony of making choices, and the anguished drudgeries of professional preparation, how could *we* (as nurses) accept with equanimity the news that now—when all our work is about to be rewarded—we are faced with the end of everything? The man with young children, the woman with a new home of her own, the newly-appointed principal, the doctor with the shiny new name plate with M.D. after his name—such people are mirrors of our aspirations, and in their dying we see evidence of our own mortality.

Because we have a tendency to closely identify with patients near our own age and social condition, it is possible that we are more likely to make errors in our attempts to help them. But why, you may ask, should this be so? Consider the following impressions.

When a thirty-five-year-old man ("Bill") looks at another thirty-five-year-old man ("John"), he may see certain similarities to himself—in the man's age, his economic condition, and his pattern of social interactions. Bill may feel that because he and John share outward similarities, both men probably share similar goals. Thus, if Bill were told that he was going to die, his primary concern might be to provide material support for his wife and two children. He may want them to continue living in the same style and he may want to make sure that his children have enough money to attend college.

If John suddenly faced death, Bill may assume that John would share his primary concerns. However, this assumption may very well be wrong; John may feel quite confident that his wife can begin where he left off and provide adequately for the family's financial support—through college and beyond. He may always have believed that neither the man nor the woman necessarily assumes the financial obligations of the family for all time, that earning the living is largely a matter of situational expedience—which changes as the circumstances change.

Thus, if a nurse so completely identifies with her patient, he may be less likely to test the accuracy of his perceptions about his patient's needs. With a patient completely different from himself the nurse may try more carefully to ascertain what he needs. Trying to determine needs is the focus of this section.

Trying to communicate a feeling without words

Human communication is beset by all kinds of obstacles that interfere with its effectiveness. For instance, people simply do not listen very carefully to one another. In school, our teachers forever admonished us to "be quiet," to "pay attention," and to participate in "discussions." However, we never really learned to pay attention or to discuss. We hear only parts of what other people say to us; we interpret their communication in terms of our own needs instead of theirs; and we become so impatient to say what *we* want to say, that we often interrupt and ignore what others are saying.

This is the situation when communication is more or less direct. How much less effective we are when our attempts at communication are indirect—when meanings are hidden or only hinted. This may occur when a topic has been surrounded by taboos—for example, when people are uncertain of how receptive others will be to discuss the topic, or when they are reluctant to put the subject into words lest their own emotions overwhelm them.

The person who is aware of his own imminent death may have needs and wants that he cannot put into words. He may be so overwhelmed by the knowledge of his dying that his feelings are confused; he needs help to sort them in order to express his wants.

Those of us who come into contact with people who are dying must develop some skill in recognizing their often unverbalized needs. To do this, we can practice developing this skill in simulated and real situations until the margin for error in assessing others' needs is substantially reduced.

All of us are currently experiencing many stresses, just in the routine of daily living, that could be alleviated by the people with whom we interact. However, virtually all of us are spared the additional stress of knowing that we will shortly die. Therefore, we can afford to take more of the risks involved in examining our behavior and making changes in our patterns of interaction.

Following is a simulated situation involving role-playing that will give us practice in learning to recognize what a person feels.

Ms. W., an attractive woman of about 35, has been told that she has an acute form of leukemia. She knows that she does not have very long to live. The woman has apparently taken the knowledge very well, since her customary mode of behavior does not seem to have changed. She holds a responsible high-level position in industry and is recognized for her competence and coolness in emergencies. Her manner is vivacious and she seems always to be laughing a little—at herself as well as at the people around her. She often makes oblique, joking references to her condition.

How do you think Ms. W. feels? Write down the feeling in a single word, if possible—such as fear, anger, shock, etc.

Mr. A. has been assigned to give nursing care to Ms. W. on this, her third admittance to the hospital. He enters Ms. W.'s room prepared to talk about her illness, if she wants, and the fact that she is dying.

Two people should assume the roles of Ms. W. and Mr. A. These are the directions for Ms. W.:

You are to *say not a word about your feeling.* You may, in any other kind of behavior, indicate that feeling, but you are not to put it *explicitly* into words. You may talk about anything else. The objective is to communicate to the "nurse" your feeling (that you have written down) without telling him directly what it is.

The directions for Mr. A. are:

Take your cues from Ms. W. in the conversation. When you think you know how she is feeling, stop the role-playing and tell her what it is.

Before Ms. W. tells Mr. A. whether or not he is right, some of the people in the rest of the class should try to guess her feeling. Briefly indicate what Ms. W. has said or done that makes you think she feels the way you say she does. After the discussion, Ms. W. can reveal her feeling and describe her words and actions which attempted to give Mr. A clues to that feeling.

If this exercise proves helpful, the whole class may pair up and act out first the patient and then the nurse in situations where the patient indirectly communicates his feeling. This role-playing need not be done in front of the rest of the class, if people prefer to work privately in pairs.

Discussion

Recently, a group of physical therapists became involved in doing the exercise. Some of them expressed surprise that they had so much difficulty in communicating how they felt, when *they* thought they were being pretty obvious. Others confessed that they just didn't know how to communicate their feelings without actually putting those feelings into words.

Those who had the opportunity to play Mr. A. seemed to appreciate the difficulty of reading people's feelings accurately and began also to focus on specific behavioral clues to others' feelings. In one such enactment, Ms. W. became irritated, and Mr. A.'s immediate response was to leave her alone until she "felt more sociable." (That was what his mother had always done to him and his sisters. Even as a four-year-old he had assessed his own need to withdraw by announcing "I'm frusterated [sic]. I think I'll go to my room until I feel better.") Mr. A. was surprised and somewhat chagrined to discover that Ms. W.'s irritation was an expression of fear that she felt would only be intensified in isolation.

Another Ms. W. smiled and smiled. Her Mr. A. thought she was cool and collected—a woman whose poise nothing could shake. *He* was shaken when everyone in the class pointed out that Ms. W.'s teeth were clenched behind all the smiling. Mr. A. was a great admirer of cool women—because his mother was a screamer.

One student playing the nurse laughingly said he could tell in advance what his Ms. W. was feeling. "Indian people are just marvelous," he said. "They accept whatever life has to offer with such fatalistic calm." It took some strong language before Ms. W. could convince him that there was nothing fatalistic or calm about what she was feeling.

Slowly the participants became aware of the more obvious pitfalls in attempting to identify people's feelings. They were:

1. Projecting their own feelings on to the other person.
2. Reading what one part of the body says and ignoring what another part is saying.
3. Being quick to identify a feeling that made them comfortable rather than searching for a feeling that disturbs.
4. Assuming the existence of certain feelings in an individual that are supposed to be "typical" of a particular group.

Learning to read patients' cues (communicating a need)

Often, the emphasis in learning to treat the dying makes the professional always the giver, and the patient always the receiver. Actually, interaction and communication with a dying person should be no different, in essence, from communication with anyone else. The essence of effective communication is that all people involved must be both givers and receivers. *Both* the patient and the nurse are critical factors in the relationship because both experience degrees of discomfort. However, though the nurse may leave with a sense of frustration, failure, or pain, she will live to try again to make successful contact with patients. The options of the dying patient are obviously more limited. Consequently, the nurse—or other health professional—must bend every effort to help the patient fulfill his potential in their relationship. The larger burden for achieving successful interaction must be assumed by the professional because he has the benefit of sustained, systematic education for making such interaction successful.

The professional needs to become sensitive to the cues patients give about their needs. When a patient says, "Come tomorrow," instead of "Don't bother me," he may be implying that tomorrow he will need help, that he will no longer be able to maintain his denial of death (from Kübler-Ross, p. 41). When the patient says, "How terrible I am; I wish my husband wouldn't visit me so often," she may be asking for help in making a decision about whether or not to discuss her feelings honestly with her husband (from Quint, pp. 218-19).

In this exercise, a class of 25 people can get some idea of the many different ways people have of communicating a single need. Take 250 small cards or pieces of paper. On half of them write the words, "Afraid and need reassurance." On the other half, write, "Need for a listener." Sit in a circle. Each person should take a packet of 5 cards that say "Afraid and need reassurance." Now, without communicating with each other in any way, write quickly, *one* idea to a card, every way you can think of to tell someone you are afraid and need reassurance. What you are indicating you need on each of these cards is someone who will *talk to you*, without expecting you to say anything. As you finish a card, throw it on the floor in the center of the circle. Give yourselves 15 minutes to write as many cards as you need.

At the end of the allotted time, someone should pick up the cards and put them in a container.

Now, each person take a packet of 5 cards marked, "Need for a listener." Again, give yourselves 15 minutes to write—one to a card— every way you can think of to let someone know that you want him to sit quietly without saying anything, and *listen to you talk* about yourself. Again, throw the cards in the center as you complete them, and have someone gather them up and put them aside in the same container with the other cards.

One person should go to the container and pick a single card. Be sure the others do not see what is written. The person should try to demonstrate the behavior on the card. The others try to decide what the person is asking for, what he is saying he needs—the need to talk or the need to listen. The first person who calls out an accurate guess should explain what led him to his conclusion. Others who guessed the same —or differently—should explain the bases of their guesses. After the others guess, the individual who demonstrated the need should tell what he was trying to communicate. Then another person should pick a card and go through the same process.

After completing this exercise, discuss generalizations you are able to make about the experience.

Discussion

One group of sixteen people who participated in such an activity were surprised to discover the great variety of ways people demonstrated a particular need. A number of participants denigrated themselves, apparently in the hope of making the listener protest the denigration and give them reassurance. For example, one person apologized for any weakness he had shown; another said his life had been worth little— "a drop in a bucket."

In startling contrast several people behaved very cheerfully and gaily, making jokes and trying to be charming. Just like the "patients" who engaged in self-denigration, this behavior also was intended to seduce the other person into responding. Here their behavior was apparently designed to enchant the listener so that he would be drawn to the patient and compelled to say "nice things."

At the other end of the behavior spectrum were two participants who acted angry and irritated in their attempts to make people talk to them and reassure them.

Some people said they would withdraw and remain silent; others said they would talk endlessly until someone got the message. Of these talkers, several were quite specific in announcing that they would talk about "something else," *not* about what they needed. One respondent would act with bravado: "Be too sure of myself." Another would act depressed. One person would "completely ignore the entire situation and hope."

The behaviors for communicating the need for someone to sit quietly and listen were also varied. Many of the expressed behaviors were exactly the same as those for getting someone to talk and reassure. Showing anger, depression, and hostility appeared, as did complete silence and excessive talking about another subject. A number of people said they would simply cry, no matter which need they had. And many said they would, directly and explicitly, indicate what it was they needed and wanted. They would say, "Don't go yet," and "Stay a while." They would ask a number of questions about themselves and their condition. One person said he would write a letter.

Many students tried unsuccessfully to tell someone they needed reassurance or a listener by "a look," or "eye contact"—behaviors that appeared in both sets of cards. They worried afterwards about how they could help a real patient effectively when all they were getting now was a beseeching look, with no specific indication of what the look meant.

Thus, it became clear to the participants that some patients would not—or could not—clearly express their needs. Consequently, it was necessary to devise some methods the nurse could use to help the patient clarify his communication.

Clarifying communication

Out of the difficulties students experienced, both in making their feelings known and in reading others' feelings, came the following exercise, designed to assist in such communication by actually providing words for the patient's use.

In role playing the situation of Ms. W. and Mr. A. (*trying to communicate a feeling without words*), Mr. A. may wish to try this technique to help himself identify the feeling Ms. W. is trying to communicate to him:

During her stay, Ms. W. complains angrily about a number of different things—the poor service, the rudeness of personnel, the noise made by other patients, and the insensitivity of her family. The nurse may have a clue that this anger is either displaced from the real object of her anger or is only a mask for another feeling. Although it is, of course, possible that conditions at this hospital were bad, it is more likely that this kind of blanket condemnation is not based on real complaints of the patient, but on the fact that she is dying—and all those other people are not. The loud talk, her anger, and her demands for attention may just be her way of announcing that she is still very much alive, that she still has the power to assert herself (from Kübler-Ross).

If Mr. W. wants to help Ms. A., he must have a clear understanding of what she is feeling. Trying to point out the obvious concern of her family for her well-being will probably not reduce her anger, nor will the observation that the only other patient in her room is too sick to make any noise, or that people generally respond politely to those who are polite to them. Acting in a reasonable or retaliatory manner cannot significantly affect anger if we are not responsive to the real causes of that anger.

To discover the real meaning of the angry behavior he is witnessing, Mr. A. first identifies the behavior and then feeds back to the patient a brief description of what he sees: "I see you feel very angry." *Then he waits for the patient to respond.* He has recognized her anger without evaluating it or the patient. The patient is free to continue the tirade or, if she wishes, give some further explanations for her feelings. She may, of course, say nothing at all.

Mr. A. then offers Ms. W. evidence that he thinks her feeling is understandable, and even justified. However, he does not go into detail about what he thinks the source of her anger is. For one thing, she may not feel ready to be completely open with him. For another, he may be mistaken in his assessment of what the source of her feeling is at this point. He merely says: "I would be angry, too, in your place." *Again he waits for the patient to respond.*

By this time, if he is listening carefully, he may get an additional bit of information about Ms. W. If she still does not respond, he may use information he knows about her from other people or from something she has said before. He feeds this bit of information back to her so that she may use it as an opening to talk more about herself: "A person as active as you have been must be furious at having to stay in bed all day." *Here, again, he must wait for the patient to respond.*

If he has been successful so far and if the patient is convinced that 1) he is listening, 2) he understands, and 3) he cares, then she may begin talking about her concerns, but not the reason for her anger. When she stops talking for a few moments, Mr. A. might prompt her: "Maybe you're thinking, 'Why did this happen to me? What have I ever done to deserve this?'" *Again he waits for the patient to respond.*

One of the most important things for the nurse to remember is that he must give the patient sufficient time to make up her mind to respond to each observation the nurse feeds back to her. If you use role-playing to practice this attempt to clarify communication, someone might hold a watch to determine how long you wait after each observation. Before the time-keeper tells you what your wait-time was, you should guess how long you waited. The chances are you will have overestimated your wait-time. We are simply not accustomed to waiting very long for anyone to respond to us. Even teachers who ask questions in the classroom rarely give children adequate time to respond before they change the question or call on someone else.

Sometimes people need time to marshall their thoughts, to get up the courage for saying something very personal, or something that has never been said before, to decide whether or not the listener is really to be trusted. If we don't leave time for such deliberation and reflection, the patient will never let us know how we can help her.

Below are a number of other responses arranged in the sequence discussed in this section. Act out any of the patient behaviors described in the other sections, and see if you can get the "patients" to become more candid about their anxieties and other feelings when you use these responses.

1. *Description of behavior:* "You wring your hands as if you're very frightened."
(Wait)
Evidence of understanding: "Being afraid is only natural."
(Wait)
Evidence of caring: "You've always believed it's important to spend a great deal of time with your children. It must be hard for you to be away from them now."
(Wait)
Helping to focus on feelings: "Maybe you're afraid because you're not sure what can be done to help you."
(Wait)
2. *Description of behavior:* "I see you're feeling very lonely and sad."
(Wait)
Evidence of understanding: "You have a right to be sad."
(Wait)
Evidence of caring: "Your friends say you're a very involved person—that you feel things deeply, and you're not afraid to show it."
(Wait)
Helping to focus on feelings: "Maybe you're thinking that this is the saddest time you've ever known."
(Wait)

Be careful to word your statements so that they may *not* easily be answered with a yes or no. If your aim is to encourage the patient to speak freely, your questions should be so worded as to need information and amplification in response. The yes or no response puts the major burden of talking back on the nurse. Since the nurse is the facilitator and *listener,* she must not assume this burden. Careful attention to the forms of her questions will keep her from falling into the trap of doing most of the talking.

Confronting fears

Although it would seem that the following exercise would be more suitable in the first section where you were trying to heighten your awareness of your feelings, it may also be appropriate now, when you are confronting the fact that you must treat dying people who are no older than you are. All the fears that we work at suppressing, at pushing out of consciousness, may now rush to the surface, no longer avoidable.

Sometimes, when we are afraid of something and never talk about our fear to other people, we begin to believe that the fear is different from anything anybody else has ever felt. We feel so alone in our fear, so isolated from other people who seem, by comparison, to be happy and comfortable. The more we feel this way, the more doubtful it seems that we can ever mention our fear to others. It might help to take a first step in acknowledging some fears about dying by checking them on a list compiled from the expressed fears of many people.

Checklist of Fears of Death and Dying

The following statements refer to *your own* death—what you are afraid of when you confront the fact that you will die:

Check here

1. I am afraid of nothingness—the end of everything.
2. I am afraid of abandoning the people who depend on me.
3. I am afraid of making those who love me unhappy.
4. I am afraid of not having time to make amends for all my sins of commission and omission.
5. I am afraid that death will be the end of feeling and thinking.
6. I am afraid of losing control over what is being done to my body.
7. I am afraid of the pain of dying.
8. I am afraid of punishment after death.
9. I am afraid of losing those I care about.
10. I am afraid of being helpless and having to depend completely on others.
11. I am afraid of dying because I don't know what happens after death.
12. I am afraid of dying before I am ready to go.
13. I am afraid of taking a long time to die.
14. I am afraid of dying suddenly and violently.
15. I am afraid of dying alone.

After checking the fears that correspond most closely to your own, find out who checked any of the numbers from 1 to 3. Have them stand together in one part of the room. Do the same with numbers 4 to 6, 7 to 9, 10 to 12, and 13 to 15. If any group has more than eight people, form a separate group of five or six of those who have checked a single item. For example, if those who are in the 1 to 3 group number eleven people, see if five or six of them have checked number 1. These people should form their own group.

Each group should sit in a small, tight circle and talk about their common fears. Try to focus on those fears that brought you together in the group, rather than talking about other fears you have. Another time you can arrange to be in a group with people who share some of your other fears.

After about ten minutes of discussion, go through the list again to form groups based on other items in the checklist. As much or as little time as you wish can be spent discussing the different fears on the list that you share with others. Perhaps you would prefer to take ten or twenty minutes of each class session over a period of a semester or a year to deal with a single item, until you have covered all the items you checked.

Discussion

Many students who engaged in this exercise expressed surprise and satisfaction at having discovered that others shared their fears—fears they thought were unique and a reflection on their maturity, courage, or good sense. This exercise seemed to change the atmosphere in the group. Their early discussions of death and dying had been characterized by intellectualization—rehashing of the descriptive data of death and dying. Discussions after this exercise were more affective, dealing with personal feelings. People seemed to trust each other more.

It may be that all of the fears held by people in the group do not appear on the list. As this becomes apparent, the list should be extended to include those fears and they should be treated the same way as the other items.

chapter eleven

———————◆◄●►◆———————

Treating the Patient
Dying in Old Age

Attitudes

Though we have a tendency to view with some equanimity the dying
and death of old people, it is still a curious fact that this apparent
equanimity does not serve to change the nature of our interaction with
the dying person. Whether the person is young or old, we seem to experience the same difficulties in developing sustained, open communication.

Perhaps it is in relation to the old person that we most need to come
to terms with our attitudes about dying. It is in confronting death in old
age that we seem to be most ambivalent. On the one hand, we reassure
each other—and sometimes even the patient himself—that he has lived a
full life and that it is time to go. On the other hand, we usually pretend
the old person is not dying. We talk about old age as the golden years,
and yet we isolate old people in "homes" or communities, where it is
certain they will stay out of the mainstream of life. Thus, we will not be
forever reminded of our own inevitable end.

Not infrequently, it is the old person who, in an atmosphere where
everyone pretends that he is not dying, tries to make his dying as comfortable as possible for the people around him. Although he may want
to talk about his impending death, he goes along with family and staff
in maintaining the pretense that he is going to get well. He talks about

everyday things with a certain amount of cheerfulness; he looks forward to the future and does not mention what is foremost in his mind.

Clarifying attitudes

Make a decision about how you feel interacting with a person who is dying. When you have completed this exercise, you might like to decide if your decision would be different if you thought of the dying people in the exercise as also being old.

Interacting with the Dying Patient

Choose from the statements below the one statement that best describes how you feel. Combine them in any way, omit parts that do not apply, and add your own words to make the statement a personal one. The important thing is that at the end you should be able to say about your statement, "This is exactly how I feel."

1. It is really not economical to spend so much time on learning how to interact with the dying. Most of our patients will be people who can respond to treatment. We need all of our limited training time to become skilled in treating those patients who are going to get better.
2. Once a diagnosis has been made and we know a patient is dying, it seems to make more sense to let other people—such as ministers and members of the family—take over the major responsibility for interacting with him. Medical personnel are more needed by the living.
3. The dying person is a living person, with the same need for good relationships with the people around him as the rest of us have. The same effort we invest in improving most of our human relationships should be expended in improving our relationship with those who are dying.
4. The best reason for learning to interact with the dying is that in the process we learn to deal with the inevitability of our own death. Those who are dying might teach us how to be less afraid and more honest about the fact of death.
5. It is morbid to think of death and dying when you're healthy and have a job to do. It is better to concentrate on living and working and enjoying life and leave the thought of dying to later, when you're old.

Ordinarily, when you do this exercise, you may keep your decision to yourself. You may just use the exercise as an opportunity to think about the various points of view at your leisure until you are satisfied that you are quite clear in your own mind about where you stand on the issue. If you decide to use the exercise this way, then there is no need to discuss it at all after you have completed the directions. However, your group may choose to discuss the various points of view, considering, perhaps, the possible social consequences of each point of view. You need not reveal your own point of view unless you choose to do so; you may like to express doubts about every point of view; you may want to point out the validities in each opinion. After all this, you may drop the issue for a while and come back to it again when you have all had the chance to think about it. In the meantime, you will continue your study of death and dying, and that may contribute to the clarification of your own point of view.

However, since you have been concerned for some time now with developing attitudes and skills for treating the dying patient, you may be ready to take a public stand on your own attitudes and values. In that case you may continue the exercise in the following way:

1. Tell the rest of your group which point of view you selected as your own. If you changed one of the opinions on the sheet, say exactly how you changed it.
2. Be prepared to state the consequences of the point of view you selected. That is, make a note of all the probable effects on patients and staff if such a point of view were hospital policy. For example, if you picked opinion number 2, you may consider such consequences as: (a) All dying patients will be put in one corner of the hospital so that they will not interfere with the routine care of other patients; (b) All dying patients will only be given minimal care for maintenance of basic comfort; (c) Only aides will care for dying patients, since the higher level skills are needed for those who are expected to recover; (d) Dying patients will be made to understand that they cannot make too many demands on the time of nurses and doctors; (e) Ministers and family members should be encouraged to take care of most of the patient's needs for interaction, since medical personnel are needed to use their professional skills with patients where there is some hope of results.

It may seem at first glance that we are reducing the above point of view to absurdity, but actually the consequences listed are merely logical outcomes of that opinion. If you cannot accept the logical consequences of what you value, then you must reconsider the stand you have taken.

When you announce your point of view, be prepared to have your colleagues point out consequences you have not thought of. Above all, you should be prepared to *defend* your point of view, using arguments that justify the anticipated consequences—or refute the logic of some of the proposed consequences.

It may be helpful to identify others in your group who agree with you. Perhaps your stand can be developed more adequately with a number of people working on it. Also, if your stand happens to be a minority point of view in your group, you may be more comfortable if you are not completely alone.

It is possible that you may be the only person with a particular point of view. In that case, the rest of the group is adjured to abide by a number of rules when comparing points of view: (a) Arguments must deal with *arguments,* and not with personalities; (b) Each point of view must be examined in terms of its consequences to people; (c) An individual must not be rejected or denigrated because he holds a particular point of view. The value of a learning situation is that it is a relatively *safe* situation, in which individuals need to feel free to state a point of view, examine it from all sides and, finally, to abandon it if they wish. In order to do this, they must be able to trust their colleagues with their doubts, their hesitations, and their half-formed thoughts. If they are attacked when they speak, they will not trust themselves in the process of learning.

No person is obligated to take a stand on an issue if he is still indecisive. Although your colleagues may point out the difficulties you may encounter if you continue to treat dying patients without being clear just how you feel about this, they may not coerce you to take a stand before you are ready to do so.

Helping the patient discover his own answers

I have always felt that telling other people how to live their lives is presumptuous. We have proverbs about the value of unsolicited advice, yet the temptation is strong to demonstrate how much more astute we are at running another person's life than he is. Parents and young children become alienated from each other over this, siblings come to blows, and aged parents are condemned, in their later years, to life styles they have never chosen.

One of the tacit stipulations the hospital society makes when a patient is admitted is that he give up control over his own life and submit to the hospital rules, regulations, and work order. The patient may find himself submitting to the arbitrary demands of individual staff members who use their own needs as the basis for their interaction with a patient. (For example, a nurse may feel she cannot spend too much time with any one

patient; therefore, she will bathe an elderly patient rather than watch
him take the slow, careful time he needs to bathe himself.)

The expectation that a patient will submit to the order of the hospital seems to reinforce a stereotype we have about old people: they are
rigid, helpless, childish, stubborn and, at best, "cute." With this stereotype in mind, it is not difficult to attempt to solve all their problems for
them—always in their own best interests, of course.

An old person has lived a long time, making his decisions and suffering
from his mistakes. Some of the prestige and stature that comes from rear-
ing a family has probably accrued to him. When a younger person—and
a stranger at that—tells him what to do, this violates his sense of self and
his sense of dignity. (With all the talk going on now about dying with
dignity, I wonder how many people consider that dignity has less to do
with the presence or absence of machines, and everything to do with
the individual's right to maintain his conception of himself as a person.)

Perhaps one reason why nurses provide solutions for people who are
troubled or perplexed is that they really know of no alternative ways to
help. Rather than watch helplessly while someone suffers, the nurse offers
help from his background and experience. However, what works for one
person is not likely to work for another person who brings to the situation different experiences, feelings and perceptions—even if that person
were willing to do what we tell them to. Perhaps if we knew how to help
a person explore his problem, try out alternative solutions, and finally
find the solution that best suits him, we could be of help without doing
violence to the patient's needs and dignity. Role-playing is a technique
that many teachers know how to use to help children develop a repertory
of skills and alternative solutions to their problems. It may sound frivolous to suggest that health-care personnel can engage in role-playing with
patients to help them solve some of their problems. But if role-playing
is not frivolous for those seriously engaged in learning to live effectively,
then it is as serious a process for those who are dying. For the dying are
not dead; they are alive and still engaged in the life-long effort to make
their interaction with others satisfying and productive.

Obviously, role-playing with a dying patient cannot take on the complicated trappings of simulation as it is often used in formal educational
situations. But the essence of this kind of simulation can be preserved in
the simple setting of a hospital bed.

Consider the following situation. See how easily it lends itself to role-
playing for identifying and practicing alternative behaviors.

> Mrs. S. is a woman of 65, who, after a year of a progressively worsening
> illness seems to have accepted with some composure the fact that she does
> not have long to live. She has a twenty-five-year-old daughter who visits

her very frequently, and who shows by her behavior that she is almost prostrate with grief at her mother's condition. Her head hangs; she always has a handkerchief in her hands that she fidgets with; she never smiles or makes eyes contact when she talks to people. She comes into her mother's room every day, sits down beside the bed, and responds with monosyllables to every effort her mother makes to start a conversation.

Usually, there are other visitors in her mother's room—friends, since there is no other family member. The talk mostly concerns casual, inconsequential matters, and the daughter does not contribute. It is as if she does not see the others or hear what they are saying. When visiting hours are over, she kisses her mother and leaves, her eyes on the floor as she makes her way down the corridor, past the nurses' station to the elevator.

Mrs. S. doesn't know what to do about her daughter; one day her concern spills over as her nurse, Ms. J., makes her comfortable for the night.

"What am I going to do about Janet?" Mrs. S. says. "She's so miserable, I'm afraid for her."

Ms. J. is tempted to tell her patient that the daughter needs a firm, no-nonsense talk to make her change her behavior. Frankly, the nurse thinks Janet is a spoiled, selfish young woman thinking only of herself, rather than her dying mother. However, Ms. J. restrains herself because she knows her patient loves her daughter dearly. The mother's worry is making her illness even harder to bear.

"Have you talked to her about her behavior, Mrs. S?" Ms. J. asks.

"I've tried, but I really don't know what to say. I can't seem to get through to her."

"Well, you know your daughter better than I do. Maybe I can help in this way. Suppose I pretend to be you, and you be Janet. I'll try to talk to you and you answer, and maybe you can get an idea of what the best thing would be for Janet."

Now the nurse playing the patient and the patient playing her daughter engage in conversation, the "patient" trying to let her daughter know how she feels, and the daughter responding. The "patient" may try first one way and then another way of helping her "daughter" understand. After the role-playing, Mrs. S. and Ms. J. discuss the alternative approaches to the daughter and the daughter's responses. One approach may be obviously more successful than another, and Mrs. S. may consider using it the next time her daughter visits or she may reject out-of-hand another approach, because she feels it is not fair to Janet. Mrs. S. may discover that she has feelings about Janet that she has never admitted before, that have become apparent in her role-playing. She may decide to tell Janet how she really feels.

After trying one or two conversations, the nurse might suggest that they reverse roles, now having Mrs. S. play herself and the nurse play her daughter. Here again, Mrs. S. may see clues, in her own and her "daughter's" responses, that enable her to decide on an effective course of action.

The point of this role-playing is that a patient, faced with a problem she cannot solve, need not submit to the advice of strangers and outsiders who may really know no more than she does. This kind of role-playing exploration in a safe setting, where one is not penalized for errors in judgment, can help a patient make a choice of the most appropriate behavior for solving her problem. Incidentally, the nurse involved in the role-playing also may gain greater understanding of her patient.

A situation similar to the one above produced a role-playing sequence that may be interesting to you. We were permitted by the participants to tape it; it is reproduced here with some key details changed to provide anonymity.

First Version of Role-playing

MRS. S. (PLAYING JANET): (Sits with her eyes downcast, twisting a handkerchief)

Ms. J. (PLAYING MRS. S.): What's the matter, Janet?

MRS. S. (PLAYING JANET): (Just shakes her head, without looking up)

Ms. J. (PLAYING MRS. S.): You've got to say something, Janet! You've got to talk to me! You can't come here day after day and just sit there! It's driving me crazy!

MRS. S. (PLAYING JANET): (In a low voice) Please. I don't mean to hurt you.

Ms. J. (PLAYING MRS. S.): Uh . . . oh . . . I'm . . . uh . . . sorry. . . .

MRS. S. (PLAYING JANET): (Puts her hand on Mrs. S.'s hand)

Ms. J.: I don't know what to say. Suddenly I can't say any more.

MRS. S.: Janet loves me. We've always been good friends. She just feels all broken up.

Ms. J.: Let me try to put myself in Janet's place. I think I understand a little more about how she feels.

Second Version of Role-playing

MRS. S. (PLAYING HERSELF): I know you love me, Janet. I know how hard this is for you.

Ms. J. (PLAYING JANET): (Sits with eyes downcast, twisting a handkerchief

Mrs. S. (playing herself): (Puts her hand on Janet's)

Ms. J. (playing Janet): (In a low voice) I feel so . . . lost. . . .

Mrs. S. (playing herself): I know. I know. But, see, I'm here. I'm with you. I love you.

Ms. J. (playing Janet): (Looks up at her mother, slowly) Oh, Mom. (Puts her hand on her mother's cheek)

Ms. J.: I realized what you were telling me. I saw you and I touched you.

Mrs. S.: I suddenly realized that it's almost as if I were gone already, to Janet. I wanted to convince her that I was still here.

One of the things Ms. J. realized was that Mrs. S. and Janet did not have enough privacy to achieve the degree of intimacy they needed if they were to find each other. With good intentions, the many friends, and even staff members, were always rushing in to make a threesome or a group; it was not always clear if they thought they were "rescuing" Janet or her mother. So Ms. J., kindly but firmly, provided mother and daughter significant blocks of time alone with each other each day. One day, Ms. J. looked into the room and saw Janet and Mrs. S. in each other's arms, crying. The nurse then knew that the patient had convinced her daughter that though she had been given a diagnosis of terminal illness she was still very much alive. Even in a hospital room, their relationship could continue to provide much for each of them—much love as well as sorrow, of learning to give and to receive, and even moments of pleasure in sharing the commonplaces of everyday living. At the end, Janet was giving her mother permission to die without blaming her and without threatening "irremedial anguish" (Kavanaugh, *Facing Death*).

section five

The Conspiracy
of Silence

chapter twelve

Telling and Knowing

The ethics and the consequences

1. Values clarification

Below are five points of view about how to tell a person that he is dying. Pick the point of view that is closest to what you believe, and change the wording until it says exactly what you think. If none of these apply, you may write a new point of view that is your own. The objective is to find a paragraph about which you can say, "This is my belief."

1. Doctors and nurses have the necessary medical expertise to know when a patient is incapable of dealing with the knowledge of his own death. The decision of whether or not to tell the patient should be left up to them. They have the best interests of the patient at heart, and it would be foolish to let the patient's disturbed emotional state interfere with what they are trying to do for him medically.

2. Under no circumstances should a person be told he is dying. The knowledge only increases everyone's suffering and discomfort—the patient's, the patient's family's, and the staff's. It is better for people to behave as if everything will turn out fine. After all, the unexpected *does* happen, so why not just keep living as usual? Then, if a person dies, he dies. That's the human condition.

3. People have a right to know *exactly* what their condition is. If a

person is dying he should be told the truth. This should be done no matter how old the person is, as long as he can understand the words life and death. Aside from the consideration that the patient might have matters he wants to take care of before he dies—the care of children, a will to be written, estranged ones to make up with—he is his own person, and no one has a right to make decisions about him in which he has no part.

4. The patient's family knows him better than anyone else, and they should know how he will react to the knowledge of his own death. If they feel that the knowledge would be too much for him, that it would make what time he had left unbearable, then the patient should not be told.

5. Ultimately, the decision of whether or not he should be told of his dying should be made by the patient. If he has never discussed the possibility of having to make such a decision, and therefore no one knows how he would really feel about it, his wishes need to be ascertained in some other way. It is the responsibility of the people who are directly concerned with the patient's welfare to develop skills for ascertaining the patient's wishes, and then acceding to those wishes.

Discussion

The objective of this exercise is to help you clarify your own values concerning the question of telling a patient he is going to die. You may realize that you are not completely sure of your point of view at this time. That is perfectly all right: perhaps now that the various points of view on the issue have been presented, you will take some time to think about it further. Therefore, you may wish later to try the values clarification exercise again and see if you are any clearer in your own mind about what you believe.

If you like, of course, you can spend some time—after you and the rest of your class have completed the exercise—to share any part of your thinking. You might like to know how the points of view are distributed in the class. Perhaps by discussing a particular point of view, your combined feelings and knowledge may help bring that point of view into sharp focus.

Above all, however, as we have noted in such an exercise in the previous section, no one should be compelled to reveal where he stands at this time, if he prefers to keep quiet until he has had more time to think about it. Nor should anyone be chastised or condemned for holding an unpopular opinion. The whole point of the exercise is to give people time and help to arrive at a point of view they can live with comfortably. Punitive pressure interferes with the freedom to think the matter through.

2. A case study

Read the following story about a patient dying of cancer. You will notice that the story is presented in italics. After each additional set of
facts you learn about the patient, stop and examine your point of view
on the desirability of letting the patient know that she is dying. There are
questions and observations at each pause to help you re-examine your
point of view in the light of the additional data.

Inevitably, at the end, the patient is dead. The family goes through
a period of grief and mourning, making their adjustments to their loss
and continuing to live their lives pretty much as before.

Would it have made much difference one way or the other if Ellen
Diser had been told or not been told that she was dying? What conclusion
do you and your colleagues come to ?

*Ellen Diser is suffering from cancer. Secondary metastases have been
discovered in her brain, though the primary site has not been located.
She cannot live for more than four or five weeks, though at this time she
is in full command of her faculties.*

At this point, knowing only these facts about Ellen Diser, would you
tell her she is dying? Defend your point of view, considering such factors
as (1) basic human rights, (2) the feelings of the doctors, nurses, other
hospital personnel, and the feelings of Ellen's family and friends. You
might also consider (3) the position of the other patients on the floor.

*Ellen Diser is forty-two years old. She has three children, an eighteen-
year-old daughter who is finishing high school, a twelve-year-old son, and
a nine-year-old son. Her husband works on the docks, loading and un-
loading ships. The family is far from affluent, but they are not uncomfortable. They have a small home with a large mortgage, yet they have
always managed to eat well, buy necessities and, from time to time, an
occasional luxury.*

*Ellen's husband Max is clearly the head of the family, making the deci-
sions lovingly but firmly. He has definite ideas about whom his daughter
should date and how late she should be permitted to stay out. He knows
what kind of work he wants his middle son to do when he gets out of
school. He dotes on his youngest child and pampers him a little.*

Suppose, after consulting with Max, Ellen's doctor decides that she is
not to be told of her impending death. Both of them feel that (1) there is
nothing she has to take care of before she dies; her husband has always
provided for everything; (2) the knowledge would only frighten her and
make her feel miserable; (3) it would interfere with their attempts to
cheer her.

Can you see any weaknesses in their reasoning? Or do you feel inclined
to agree with them? Justify your answer.

Ellen's relationship with her children has always been a good one. She is a conscientious mother, and has provided a clean home, good cooking and concern for the health and safety of her family. When the children needed help with schoolwork, she did what she could; when they cried, she comforted them; when they wanted toys and clothes, she bought them what she could and explained when she couldn't.

It seems to be going along all right, doesn't it? The relationships are comfortable, and no unnecesssary stress has been introduced. The doctor's decision has apparently been the correct one.

It is true that Ellen has never discussed any subjects of great significance with her children. Her parents never did with her, either, and she feels she is none the worse for it. Concerns about sex, for example, have a way of resolving themselves without discussion. Anyway, she knows she has good children, and she isn't overly concerned about their future.

At this point, can you see any reason why Ellen might need to know that she is going to die? How about her children? Do you think *they* might need to feel free to talk about the subject with her?

The patient in the next bed envied Ellen her family. They came often, bringing her small gifts and keeping up a constant cheerful chatter, telling her about the things happening to them at home, at school, and at work. Ellen always spoke cheerfully and smiled at their funny stories. They were so good with each other.

Have your doubts been allayed about the decision? The cheerful good humor is much better for everyone than the anger and sadness they would feel about dying. Of course, the family must feel badly about losing their mother, but they have each other to grieve with and to console. At least they are making their mother's last days as pleasant as possible.

Sometimes, however, Ms. Schultz wondered why Ellen seemed so sad the moment her family left each day. A couple of times it almost seemed as if she breathed a sigh of relief as soon as she was alone.

How do you feel about the situation now? Of course, maybe Ellen is just a little tired after her family leaves, and is relieved to have a few hours to relax without company. And her sadness can easily be understood: it is, after all, no fun to be in a hospital, with people doing all kinds of unpleasant things to you.

Ms. Schultz is able to walk up and down the corridor outside their room. She often stops to chat with other patients and with the staff members at the nurse's station. One day, she learned that Ellen was dying. Of course, she was resolved not to mention this to Ellen. She knew she could keep a secret when it was necessary.

What about Ms. Schultz's needs? What is happening to her as a result of the decision to keep Ellen's condition from her? Is there something owed to Ms. Schultz in this regard? Or needn't anyone be concerned about her, since Ellen and her problem are no business of Ms. Schultz, who is, after all, a total stranger?

Ms. Schultz, who had been friendly with Ellen since her admission to the hospital, began to feel uncomfortable in her presence. She found herself laughing a lot, and her laugh sounded strange in her ears. Under other circumstances she might have asked a neighbor in the next bed if she felt all right, or remarked aloud that she didn't look very happy, yet she found herself unable to say such things to Ellen. She found herself talking more and more to her own visitors behind a drawn screen, and leaving the screen around her bed until she went to sleep. It was easier to avoid Ellen than to keep looking into her eyes and pretending.

Do you have any thoughts about how Ellen Diser may now feel about Ms. Schultz's behavior?

Actually, Ellen is quite content to be left alone when her family is not around. She prefers to do without the constant strain of cheerfulness. Also, the pain is becoming more persistent. The medicine doesn't seem to help as much as it did at first.

Finally, at two o'clock one morning, Ellen died in her sleep. Her family learned the news by a telephone call from the night nurse, John Forster, as he had been instructed to do by the physician in charge. Although John had expected Ellen to die soon, and he made a point of checking on her regularly, she died when she was alone. For a while, the thought of this disturbed him, until he forgot about it in the pressures of his work. When he called, John suggested the family should go to the hospital morgue for a last look at Ellen's body before they made arrangements for her burial. Afterward, they cried and consoled each other, saying at least they had made her last days cheerful.

Ms. Schultz put Ellen out of her mind. When she did remember her fleetingly once in a while, a slight frown crossed her face.

How would you remember Ellen—if you were John Forster, or Ms. Schultz, or her physician, her husband, her child?

Children and knowing

Elisabeth Kübler-Ross suggests that children who are isolated from hospitals and death have no language to talk about death. Consequently, they rely on symbolic language—both non-verbal and verbal—to communicate their feelings and thoughts. The nurse who does not understand the meaning of a symbolic communication may find it more productive to merely listen, rather than to probe for meaning and try to push the child into talking more plainly. As with older patients, the important thing seems to be to demonstrate caring, by touching, by holding, by *being there,* until the patient feels able to begin to talk and finds the words to do so.

It is likely that children have more words to talk about death than we think they do. There is much sentiment in our culture about protecting children from knowledge of the harsh realities of living. So pervasive is this sentiment, that we often cut off meaningful communication between the generations. Children are often aware of the realities, yet because they are denied the benefit of our experience and assistance, they often perceive those realities through a distorting mist of fear and misconception.

In the area of race relations, for example, adults are fond of asserting that "children have no prejudices." Only a passing observation will almost invariably reveal clearly identifiable prejudices against racial groups, religious groups, different nationalities, as well as sex-group prejudices. Yet even teachers seem to think that the overt racial hostility of high school students and adults somehow springs full-blown into being at that point where the hostility turns into physical violence. And most adults still seem to think that small children are not concerned with sexual stereotypes.

Similarly, we often delude ourselves into believing that children do not think about death. Actually we may arrange our life to avoid knowing just what children *are* concerned with. When someone in the family is dying, we either send the children away, or do not discuss the matter in front of them, or actually refuse to talk to them about it. Certainly hospitals—where so many people die—have rules that keep children from coming to visit.

When we are finally forced by the pressures of reality to give some sign of recognition to the child that a person is dying or is dead, we speak in euphemisms and use other evasions, so that the child is never quite sure of what exactly has happened. It is not inconceivable that what we believe is a developmental perception of dying—the idea that the person has "gone on a trip"—is actually taught to the child by adults. Certainly the dead person as an angelic figure looking down from the sky is adult-inspired fantasy.

1. Sharing the thoughts and feelings of children

When a child is dying in the hospital, it may be that the strangeness of the hospital situation and the determined avoidance of his family and the hospital staff are responsible for the child's reluctance to speak realistically about dying—rather than his supposed "lack of words" or "inability" to conceive of death. In fact, children apparently *do* deal with the idea of death and dying in direct ways when given the opportunity.

The twelve-year-old who wrote the following poem was one of six children in a class of twenty-eight who wrote about death without being directed to do so.* This child is afraid of dying. She has had a personal experience with death, and she has not forgotten it. However, she thinks it is better to shut out the awareness of death "and think of happy things." Who else, besides her teacher, knows about her fears and her struggle to deny? I wonder, also, what more is being done to help her confront the fact of death and come to terms with it.

The Rain

It makes me sad to think of all those who are dead
And everytime it rains they pop into my head
The rain represents all my tears
And also makes me think of my fears

It makes me think of Caren's dad
Who was always happy never sad
And then one bright and sunny day
The Lord came and took his life away

It makes me think of funerals too,
The rain makes me oh so blue.

The wind that splashes all rain,
gives me sort of an emotional pain.

But the rain, you really must think
Mustn't always make your eyes pink

And when it starts to pour
Lock and shut your front door
And think of happy things.

by Sharon Way

Another one of the six children goes from a shocking picture of death to peace in heaven. Somehow, the horror creeps through the sentimentality and denial.

The stiffened body lies motionless
Upon the cold, damp ground.
He looks upon her loveliness
But does not make a sound

To think that God should take a life
And destroy astounding beauty,
Inside he realizes that the death of his wife
Must be an unpleasant duty.

He's sure of one thing in his heart
That now he knows the deceased

---

* The children were pupils of Ms. Merril Stup, a Philadelphia teacher.

Will go into heaven to be with God
And then shall Live in Peace.

by Carol Zimme

The idea that laughing is better than crying, and that it is necessary to "cheer up" a grieving person is a point of view that filters through to the next child from our culture. But what disastrous results!

What is striking about this story is the absence of talking by the bereaved. There is crying and remembering, but no talking. One wonders if Ira ever had a chance to talk about his grandfather before he put pen to paper.

> On March 16, 1972, my grandfather (Pop-Pop) died at his house two blocks away from us. It was drizzling when my mother called my two sisters and I from my grandparents' house. My oldest sister answered the phone and when she hung up later she was crying. I suspected he was dead so I sniffed a little then I let it all pour out. After that my middle sister just looked at my oldest sister and I crying. 20 minutes later (approximately) I ran out of "juice". My middle sister and I then just watched my oldest sister cry. I didn't think she'd ever stop! I don't blame her for crying so much since we all loved him so dearly. (I can still remember him taking us to Woolworth's parking lot on Sundays and we would try and find pennies. He would throw the pennies and we would say we found them.) I decided to try and cheer her up by saying a funny line or two, but she kept right on crying. So I turned on the T.V. show "Me and the chimp" and she started to laugh. I felt good knowing she felt good, but the show was over by the time she was laughing hard.
>
> The next Saturday was the funeral and it was raining. I saw my Pop-Pop in the coffin and my uncle was really crying. Worse then my sister! I didn't cry because I ran out the other day. This time both sisters were crying. When we left the burial grounds it was pouring rain. My oldest sister went hysterical in the car when my dad started the motor. She screamed, "Dad stop the car! We can't leave Pop-pop here! Dad!" So now every time it rains I think of that one time.
>
> by Ira Wolins

In the following poems by children, rain brings neither new growth nor cleansing, but pain and death. All the doggerel we feed children about April showers, and flowers, and sparkling drops on the windowpane doesn't seem to have registered with these children. How many others are too timid to break through our defensive shields?

> Rain brings pain to many people.
> Deaths on highways
> Accidents in skyways.

> Many people dying day by day,
> Other people left in a very sad way,
> And many people are left astray,
> Rain creates problems in its own funny way.

by Celia Uchitel

Rain represents tears to some children, perhaps a symbol of grieving that is never finished. In the two poems that follow, the words do *not* represent "emotion recollected in tranquility." On the contrary, the crying seems to go on and on with bitterness unresolved and sadness undiminished.

What Is Rain?

> Rain is something very awful
> And soon I'll tell you why
> It can be good, too
> Nevertheless, it makes me cry
>
> Roses are brought from rain
> And sadness is brought, too
> It stops me from doing what I want,
> And leaves me with nothing, whatever to do
>
> Rain makes me think
> Of a time that I'll always remember
> It was a time that my sister was told that she'll die
> *That* was in December
>
> See, she developed cancer
> And died, not so far away
> That terrible day that she left us
> February 14th was the day
>
> So whenever rain starts pouring down
> I can't do anything, but think, and sob
> That the doctors tried to save her
> But they sure did a lousy job

by Mimi Kohn

Rain

> He's gone now,
> I guess we really didn't care.
> He left without us even knowing he was there.
> He liked the rain,
> I don't know why.
> I guess he just liked,
> the color of the sky.

When all the rain
would come pouring
down and he would
love to watch it clinging
to the window pane.
He would get a feeling
of comfort in his bones.
Why did he have to go,
when. . . . . drip, drip oh no
not now he must be
up there now he's crying.
I can feel it.
I'll think of him every time it rains.
Well, goodbye now
pop, I wish you
would stop you
know I can't stand
to see a grown man
cry.

by Susan Thomas

Can anyone after reading what these children have written believe that, should one of them contract a serious illness, he could be distracted from the truth by evasions, lies, and pampering? At some point, we simply must admit that our silence with children and with adults is similarly motivated. Perhaps the skills and sensitivities we develop for interacting with dying adults can be equally useful in treating dying children.

2. Remembering from our own childhood

A student recalled an experience she had concerning the shooting of President Kennedy when she was eleven years old. When someone told her he had been shot, she shrugged her shoulders and observed that she was sure the best doctors would be found for him, and that he would surely recover. When he died, she was left with a feeling of anxiety and guilt. She knew, of course, that one could not cause the death of another by indifference, or by saying what she did. Nevertheless, some vague anxiety remained that she had somehow contributed to his death.

"I stayed glued to the television set for the whole funeral, because I felt somehow obligated," she said. "Later, a friend of mine said, 'See, even a President can die—even with the best doctors,' and this made me feel worse. For years, every time something happened to the Kennedy family, it really depressed me."

Today this student worries about the death of her mother who is neither old nor ill.

Do you have similar memories of the death of someone famous, or someone close to you? Sit apart from everyone else and close your eyes. Become again the child you were: six years old, ten years old, or eleven or twelve. Imagine that your teacher has asked you to write a poem or a composition on one of the following topics. Pick a topic, then take an hour to write a poem or a composition recalling some experience with death: the feeling, the atmosphere, the person, or anything else about that experience that the topic suggests:

Rain
Darkness
The Dream
The Endless Space
Winter Cold
The Tree Without Leaves
Footsteps in the Dark
The Giant

When you have finished your poem or composition, you might like to read it aloud to the other people in your group. After you have heard a number of them, you may get some idea of the extent of awareness and concern that children have with dying and death. Consider what you as children would have liked to have had from the adults in your lives. A chance to talk? Some encouragement to ask a question? An explanation?

What do you think children today would like to have from you?

chapter thirteen

———◄●►———

Levels of Awareness

Much data about dying indicate that dying patients usually know they are dying, even if they have not been told so directly.* Unless there is open communication about dying between the patient and the people around him, much suffering is caused by the attempt to maintain the fiction that the patient will survive.

The problems surrounding the question of *how* to tell a patient he is dying are not being solved. This remains such a difficult task that many doctors continue to avoid it (often managing to do so only by avoiding the patient). Nurses appear to have an easier way to avoid the task: they maintain that the job of informing a patient is the doctor's, that the nurse says nothing without the doctor's express permission. Since the doctor must rationalize his avoidance behavior, he often maintains that it is not in the best interests of the patient to be told, or that his family doesn't want him to be told. And so it goes.

Considering the objective data on the one hand and the doctors' feelings of discomfort on the other, it seems as if the nurse must reassess her professional position on this matter. If she is with a dying patient for long periods of time, she has vital information on which to base the decision to tell him the truth. Also, the appropriate moment for telling

---

* The levels of awareness used in this chapter are defined by Glazer and Strauss in *Awareness of Dying*, Aldine Publishing Co., Chicago, 1965.

him—or at least responding to his questions—may come and go when no doctor is present. It seems a disservice to the patient to postpone responding to his questions—and to his needs—because the people who are identified as appropriate respondents are either psychologically or physically absent.

A person who gives information must know how much the other person already knows. If the receiver knows too little, the new information may not be understood—the learner may not be able to use the additional information. If the receiver knows too much, he may resent the giver's implication that he *needs* the information, and so may refuse to engage in further communication.

Let us illustrate this fact with an example from the problem of letting a patient know he is dying. Suppose that a patient has no idea he is suffering from a terminal illness (closed awareness). To say to such a patient, "You have three months to live," can be a brutal shock, and may unnecessarily tax the patient's psychological resources, not giving him the time he needs to absorb the information at his own rate of speed. Consequently, he may actually shun awareness of this information and continue to live as if he were not dying.

On the other hand, when a patient who knows he is going to die (open awarenesses) asks, "How long do I have?" he seems ready to learn that he has less than three or four months. But if he is told, "There are still tests to make and we don't know what effect the treatment will have," he may turn in distrust from the one who gives him too little information, and never again ask such an important question.

1. Determining the Patient's Level of Awareness

Here is an exercise that may help you become skillful in determining the patient's level of awareness of his own dying and the level of his specific knowledge about his illness. Read the following conversations one at a time. After you have read one, note whether you think it reveals: (1) the patient does not know that he is dying, (2) the patient has some suspicion that he is dying, (3) the patient knows that he is dying, but he is pretending not to know, (4) the patient knows he is dying and is ready and willing to talk about it.

When everyone has decided what the conversation reveals, discuss the bases of your decision and try to identify the clues that led to your decision. See if you can understand why some of you thought the patient was revealing one level of awareness, and other students another. Finally, can you say that your discussion does result in a fairly general agreement? If not, perhaps reading Glaser and Strauss's book, *Awareness of Dying,* might give you some additional information that you need.

CONVERSATION A

DOCTOR: There is an operation we can do to take away the pain.

PATIENT: To take away the pain?

DOCTOR: Yes. It will make you more comfortable. You'll be able to get around a little more.

PATIENT: My family gets so upset when I'm in pain. I hate upsetting them.

DOCTOR: This operation should help the pain.

CONVERSATION B

PATIENT: (to the nurse who has come into the room) Oh, Miss Jones, my husband and I were just planning a trip to the West Indies next spring.

NURSE: (smiling) I've never been to the West Indies.

PATIENT: Neither have we. I've never been on a boat—ship? I never know which word to use.

NURSE: Neither do I.

PATIENT: Anyway—it's a cruise. I'm really looking forward to it!

NURSE: As pleasant as this is, I have work to do. Can't chit chat like some people I know! (Leaves)

CONVERSATION C

PATIENT: Some days I feel worse, and I almost think it's the end. But maybe it's just my imagination.

NURSE: Are you asking me?

PATIENT: Asking you what?

NURSE: If it's your imagination.

PATIENT: Oh, some days I feel worse. But some days I feel better.

CONVERSATION D

PATIENT: (crying)

NURSE: You keep crying all the time. It just makes you feel sicker.

PATIENT: I just can't help it. I can't seem to be able to stop.

NURSE: How do you think it makes your family feel? You're making it harder for them.

PATIENT: I know, I know. I don't want to make it harder for them.

2. Providing Opportunity for Changing Awareness

After you have discussed the clues that helped you decide how aware the patient was of his impending death, you may want some help in developing ways of assisting the patient to go from one level of awareness to another—toward open awareness and, ultimately, toward open awareness with peace.

Following are a number of suggested responses to each one of the above conversations that might be useful in changing the patient's level of awareness. The choice of whether or not to change is left to the patient in each case. The nurse—or other member of the health care team —merely presents a window through which the patient may see an alternative to his present behavior. Whether or not he finds such an alternative must be left to him. In the final analysis, the nurse's diagnosis of his awareness and of his need may be wrong. What she says may propel him into even greater isolation running from someone who obviously does not understand him. Trying to force awareness or pushing a patient to behave differently is an unwarranted interference with his freedom, no matter how well-intentioned that interference may be.

Write each one of the following conversational openings on a separate card and shuffle the cards. *Do not number the items.* Then, in small groups, have each person draw a card and try to match it to the appropriate conversation. Each person should explain how the suggested gambit on the card can lead the patient from the level of awareness he seems to reveal toward a more open awareness.

Do not read the discussion following the list of conversational openings until you have completed the exercise.

1. This operation should stop the pain, but it won't cure.
2. Do you think if you talked to them about your illness, it would help them understand?
3. Do you think you'll be well enough for such a trip?
4. You're planning a long way ahead.
5. That's such a long time from now. Why don't you tell your husband about the Thanksgiving party we're planning on this floor?
6. What does the end mean to you?
7. What is it you feel when you say you feel worse?
8. I'll sit here beside you for a while; maybe it will help you feel better.

Discussion

Conversational window #1 is suitable for Conversation A. It offers an item of information—*it won't cure*—but in such a way that the patient need not recoginze its full import if he chooses. Although it is clearly stated that the suggested operation will not cure the illness, the patient may still feel this is not the whole story—that cure may still be possible after the problem of pain is eliminated. On the other hand, if the patient wishes he may pursue the matter further, clarifying in his own mind the purpose of surgery that does nothing but offer comfort.

Conversational window #2 also can be used with the patient in Conversation A. This is an alternative suggested in the form of a question to encourage the patient to give some thought to the reasons for her family's "upset." The question implies that at least part of the family's upset stems from other causes than the patient's pain. What those other causes might be could be revealed in the course of more open communication—an openness that might be initiated by the patient. The statement also implies that the patient has knowledge about his illness that he could share with his family. Even though the family probably has the same knowledge, the patient's open admission that he also knows may ease the tension and discomfort for all concerned.

Conversation B presents a difficult problem: How can the nurse give the patient an opportunity to come out of a complete lack of awareness without being brutally open? It would seem at first glance that almost anything that does not go along with the deception is too revealing and coercive. However, some conversational windows do occur to me that might be useful.

Conversational item #3 poses a question that the patient may or may not choose to consider. She may ignore it, or not take it seriously, or she may stop and ask for additional information: "Don't *you* think I'll be well enough?" As fearful as she may sound, if the patient does ask this question, she is probably ready to receive some information.

Conversational window #4 also leaves the choice of pursuing the matter to the patient. "You're planning a long way ahead," may easily be interpreted as a non-committal response to any long-range planning. However, it may be interpreted as a cautionary response: Don't plan so far in advance. If the patient is ready to learn more about her condition, she may ponder this warning and then ask a question.

The #5 conversational window is a little more direct. It actually says: Plan for next week, not next year. Again the nurse resists playing a deception game. She also implies a caution against planning for the distant future. Most important, perhaps, she focuses the patient on present living. It is likely that over a period of time the cumulative effects of many such cues will gradually raise the patient's consciousness to the point where she asks for additional information.

In Conversation C the patient chooses to ignore the nurse's cue. The nurse says: "Are you asking me (if it's only your imagination that you are dying)?" This is an open offer to tell the patient what she almost seems to know. But the patient backs away from the offer, preferring for the moment to live with suspicion rather than certainty. This is her right. If she prefers never to accept the fact that she is dying, she must be left free to die without everyone talking openly about her own death.

There are other approaches that might be useful to patients who only suspect that they are dying, seeming sometimes to move closer to awareness and then veering off to avoid coming too close. Conversational window #6 questions the patient on what has just been said. Should the patient not want to reveal her feelings about dying, she may say quite directly, "I don't want to talk about it." Or, less directly, "Oh, I don't know. It's just an expression." On the other hand, she may welcome the opportunity to begin to talk about dying, even though she may not immediately talk about her own dying.

Window #7 also encourages the patient to respond. It picks up on something the patient has said about his own condition, and encourages him to talk more about this. The chances are that he will be able to focus in on symptoms at first, which is something that most people are quite willing to do. In the course of describing his symptoms, the patient may reveal his feelings and begin to speak more directly about dying.

Obviously, windows #6 and #7 cannot be used while the nurse is in a hurry to leave. *The chair beside the patient's bed must be used.* Unfortunately, many nurses and doctors would not dream of sitting down beside their patient, leaning forward, and preparing to listen to the responses to these questions. Occasionally, a doctor may sit down to *tell* a patient something, but sitting down to listen is not generally considered to be part of patient care.

Conversational window #8 deals with a situation where the patient knows that she is dying. The chances are that she has found out fairly recently and is still suffering some shock from the knowledge. Her constant crying probably comes partly from fear and even terror at the prospect of what lies before her. It would seem that she could profit most from putting some of these feelings into words. By talking about what she thinks is happening to her and beginning to ask specific questions, she may receive answers which will allay some of her worst fears.

Admonishing the patient to, in effect, stop indulging herself and to consider the feelings of her family ignores her real need. In addition, there is an implied moral censure that merely adds to her burden. The nurse's idea of the proper way to die should *never* be imposed on the patient. The patient must be helped to find her own way of dying, a way that is consistent with everything she is as a person.

The patient who is crying may just need some time to finish the crying before she is ready to talk. In this case conversational window #8 may be helpful. It is an announcement that the nurse understands her need to cry and is ready to listen to her and comfort her whenever she is ready to talk and be comforted. Perhaps the first or second time the nurse sits down for five minutes, the crying goes on and nothing else happens, and the nurse must leave to take up other duties. However, it must not be supposed that the time spent at the patient's bedside is wasted; one of the things it does for the patient is give her time to trust the intentions of those around her. Before she shares her feelings with the nurse, she needs some assurance that, once a certain amount of dependence develops (and sharing feelings *does* create dependence on the empathy and acceptance of the other person) she will not then arbitrarily be abandoned to shift for herself. She needs to know that at least one person is ready to stop with her and take the time to respond to a need that is not specifically medical.

At this time in our history, it is generally agreed that the nurse is not the one who should assume the responsibility for informing the patietn that he is dying. However, one day the nurse may be responsible; perhaps doctors may be happy to be relieved of the burden. If nurses are willing to prepare themselves to feel reasonably comfortable in speaking openly with the dying patient, then they may hasten the day when they take the leadership responsibility. Any group that knows how to do something cannot indefinitely be kept from doing it in a society where there is desperate need for the skill.

chapter fourteen

Simulation: Trying to Function with Variations in Awareness

Justifying simulation

It seems almost frivolous to suggest game-playing for the purpose of becoming skillful in dealing with death. However, simulation is proving to be a valuable aid to skill development in many areas, including at least one that has far less to recommend it—war.

The objectives of simulation are rather obvious. Short of engaging in the real situation, the individual becomes involved in observing the behavior of others, becoming aware of his own attitudes, facing alternatives, making choices, and learning what the consequences are of his decisions. The beauty of simulation is that it is safe. Errors are never a matter of life and death; and one can always come back to play again, utilizing what he has learned in previous games to avoid mistakes and even to win. The individual thus develops a background of knowledge and a repertory of refined skills in a sheltered situation, before he goes into the real world to use that knowledge and those skills. Thus simulation is not a substitute for life experience; it is merely an opportunity to prepare for it.

The game

This simulation is a very simple one that deals with essentials of observation and decision-making. It requires no complicated equipment or

153

special space, and can be played with as few as two people or as many as ten, if you can find counters small enough to fit so many on a simple checkerboard square.

On ordinary 3 × 5 *white* index cards, write the following list of patient items, one item to a card:

Patient items

1. You don't want your sixteen-year-old daughter to know you are dying. Stay where you are.
2. You tell the nurse that you know you are going to die. Go forward three spaces.
3. You ask a friend to bring you an application blank for enrolling in college courses next fall. Go back three spaces.
4. You cry and tell the nurse that you worry about leaving your small children who are so helpless and need their mother. Go forward one space.
5. *Make a choice.* You may go forward two spaces, but first you must tell your patient's aunt that her niece will be all right.
6. If you lied in any one of the last three moves, go back five spaces. The person to whom you lied has found out the truth.
7. You overhear a conversation between two aides and learn that you have been deceived: you are going to die. Go forward one space.
8. You have learned by accident that you are going to die. You decide to pretend that you don't know the truth. Go back four spaces.
9. If you pretended you didn't know you were going to die in the last three moves, go back two spaces. You have discovered that your husband is agonized trying to decide whether or not to tell you.
10. You are furious because the only answers you receive are evasive ones. You finally shout at the doctor, "Nobody will tell me anything. Nobody will talk to me!" Go forward three spaces.
11. The doctor tells you that you have multiple myeloma. You say to him, "I want to know exactly what that is." Go forward four spaces.
12. You feel fine today so you decide to go home immediately. Go back three spaces.
13. You tell the doctor you'll keep on your diet if he promises you will be able to go home for Christmas—eleven months from now. Go back three spaces.
14. You tell your mother that she's never really loved you and that she needn't pretend to care by coming to visit you. Stay where you are.
15. *Make a choice.* You may go forward one space, but first you must not reveal that you suspect people aren't telling you the truth about your condition.

16. If you kept your suspicions to yourself in the preceding move, go back three spaces. Everyone around you suspects that you know.

17. *Make a choice.* You may go forward two spaces, but first you must tell a co-worker of yours that you expect to be on the job in a few weeks.

On ordinary 3 × 5 *colored* index cards, write the following list of nurse items, one item to a card:

Nurse items

1. You feel terrible that the patient had to go back three spaces because she is hopeful and planning for the future. Go back three spaces.

2. You tell the patient not to worry—to concentrate on getting well. Go back three spaces.

3. If you lied in any one of the last three moves, go back five spaces. The person you lied to knew the truth all along.

4. *Make a choice.* You may go forward two spaces, but first you must tell a co-worker of yours to keep the patient's prognosis a secret from him.

5. You are annoyed when an aide suggests to you that the patient suspects he is dying. Go back four spaces.

6. You sit down at the patient's bedside and tell him you have a little time to talk. Go forward two spaces.

7. You are searching to find a way to tell the doctor that you think he should be honest with the patient. Go forward two spaces.

8. You tell the doctor you think he should respond openly to the patient's questions. Go forward five spaces.

9. You decide that it is the doctor's responsibility to let the patient learn about his dying. You continue to pretend the patient will get well. Go back five spaces.

10. *Make a choice.* You may go forward four spaces, but first you must say nothing to the other patients in your hospital unit about the patient who died during the night.

11. If you kept quiet when you should have talked in the last two moves, go back four spaces. The people you didn't talk to are made more anxious by your silence.

12. You answer "yes" to the patient's question, "Am I going to die?" Go forward four spaces.

13. You tell your supervisor how grateful the patient is for your honesty. Go forward four spaces.

14. You lash out in anger at the student nurse because she cried when she heard the patient was dying. Go back three spaces.

15. You asked a student to answer the patient's light because you don't like his constant complaints about the hospital. Go back two spaces.

16. You say nothing when the patient says, "If only I could be with my family on Christmas, I would die content." Go back one space.
17. You encourage the patient to talk about the worries she has and the provisions that must be made to care for her small children. Go forward three spaces.

Directions

1. Decide which players are patients and which are nurses. (Since you play as individuals, there need not be an even number in each role.)
2. Use an ordinary checkerboard and—for two players—one black checker and one red checker. (You may use different colors of cardboard counters or small metal toys. Each player must have his own identifiable piece for moving around the board.)
3. Shuffle each stack of cards.
4. Put the stacks of cards to one side of the board.
5. Decide the order of playing. As you play, alternate a nurse player and a patient player.
6. The first player turns up a card from his stack (Nurse or Patient as it applies) and reads it aloud. He follows the direction, moving his playing piece from the CLOSED-AWARENESS square in the direction indicated below:

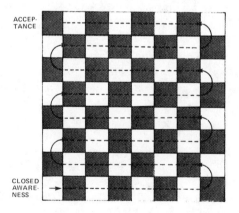

7. When all the cards have been drawn, re-shuffle them and go on playing.
8. The objective is to arrive at ACCEPTANCE. The first player who does so wins.

If you like, you may add additional stacks of cards for players representing members of the patient's family and other staff members. It is conceivable that any one player may reach the stage of acceptance of death before others do. An aide may do so while a physician is still essentially denying; a patient may do so even if the nurse is still avoiding the topic.

With a larger number of players, you might use a large playing surface. It is easy to rule squares on a sheet of poster board or a length of wrapping paper and use that instead of a checkerboard. With such a large surface, you might make the game more interesting by writing additional directions on some of the squares. When your playing piece lands on one of these squares, follow the directions. Below are some suggestions, which may be supplemented by your knowledge and imagination. The directions on the squares deal primarily with conditions in the environment that encourage or impede progress toward acceptance, rather than with the behavior of the patient or the nurse.

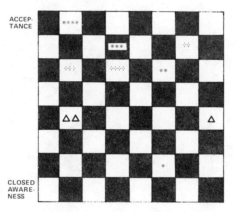

* The six-bed room interferes with the intimate atmosphere you need to talk about death. Go back two spaces.

** You are always two nurses short on a shift, so you have barely enough time to do the required work. Go back two spaces.

*** The hospital policy states that visiting is permitted only during specific hours. Go back one space.

**** Every patient is sedated so he will sleep all night. Go back three spaces.

† No children are permitted in your hospital unit. Go back three spaces.

†† Patients are not permitted to have their personal belongings—such as pictures, typewriters, etc. Go back two spaces.

††† Every nurse in your hospital unit is afraid of the supervisor who insists that all rules be obeyed and all procedures followed exactly. Go back three spaces.

†††† Doctors never come to health team meetings. Go back three spaces.

* All dying patients are moved—by hospital policy—to one end of the hospital unit. Go back four spaces.

** Student nurses have no course work in interacting with dying patients. Go back four spaces.

section six

The Process of Observation

chapter fifteen

The Rationale for Systematic Observation

Specific objectives

Instruments for systematic observations of behavior have been used in the field of education for a long time. They have proved useful for helping observers to identify and record specific behaviors that contribute to effective or ineffective interaction between people—teachers and pupils, student teachers and supervisors and, occasionally, administrators and teachers. One objective of systematic observation has been:

1) To give feedback to the one observed and so refine his awareness of exactly what he is doing when he is in a classroom.

It is not unusual, for example, for a teacher to insist that she wants her pupils to respond to questions. She may believe that with the variety of questions and the various levels of knowledge to which the questions address themselves, every question might reasonably be expected to produce a response. However, her pupils are not responding to her questions; she finds herself almost invariably giving them the answers, or berating them for not doing their work. When asked, she attributes their lack of responses to the "fact" that they are "slow," or "non-verbal," or "lazy." If she works with black or Puerto Rican or Chicano children, she may feel particularly justified in such an evaluation of them, since it is quite consistent with her preconceptions about what such children are like. Unless she can be convinced that there is something about the way she is interacting with the children that is inhibiting their responses, she will continue to maintain her low level of expectation about their ability. Having such a minimal expectation, she will naturally teach only the bare minimum of the curriculum. Her children will consequently learn very little, and her low expectations will have been justified. *Her own behavior will have caused the children's lack of response, but she will not realize this.*

However, when an observer can point to an observation record that shows unmistakably that every question the teacher asks is followed after a one-second interval by the teacher herself giving the information, it is difficult for the teacher to persist in her delusion that she is giving pupils an opportunity to answer questions. It is almost impossible for her to avoid admitting what she is doing.

2) Another objective of systematic observation has been to help the person observed focus on the consequences of specific behaviors in an interactive situation, so that he may adopt those behaviors that produce the desired responses, and discontinue those that produce unwanted responses. After his level of awareness has been raised, his next step is to change his behavior.

When a teacher responds to a pupil's expression of feeling with what he believes is accepting behavior, he may be disturbed and confused to discover that the pupils seem always either to become hostile or to withdraw into silence. In talking about this experience, he reports that he appreciates the pupils' feelings and really wants them to feel free to express them openly in the classroom. He may conclude that his pupils are "naturally reticent," or that they do not like him because he is white or Black, or that the generation gap is simply unbridgeable.

On the other hand, the systematic observer of this teacher's behavior is in a position to record that the so-called accepting behavior is invariably the question, "Why do you feel this way?" Since this is the kind of question that adults are always asking children, the observer might also have thought that it was a perfectly good question, encouraging continued open responses and contributing to an atmosphere of acceptance between teacher and pupils. However, since the answer to this question is never the desired one, both observer and teacher must conclude that some alternative response to a pupil's expression of feeling would be more desirable. The teacher is almost compelled to change his behavior.

3) The ultimate objective of any observation of teacher behavior is, of course, to help the pupils make the most of their learning opportunities, to help them feel good about themselves and their efforts, and to help them interact productively with other people.

The child who needs praise and recognition of his efforts to achieve may falter and fail with a teacher who accepts his work without comment. The child whose understanding of ideas is developed through his own questioning and commenting can be lost with a teacher who does all the talking in the classroom. Through heightened awareness and changes in her own behavior, the teacher provides an opportunity for the children to get the most out of the situation in which they find themselves.

Similarly, the student teacher in her relationship with her supervisor is more likely to become a competent professional if her supervisor's behavior does not intervene to block her progress. She should be able to take advice without becoming either hostile or defensive if her supervisor becomes aware of the danger of certain supervisory behaviors and learns to avoid them. She will feel free to use what she has learned in college without excessive fear of failure, if the behavior of the supervisor communicates acceptance and support. She should see herself as worthwhile, even though she must ask questions and admit ignorance of some aspect of her work. Observational techniques that make the supervisor aware of the student's behavior and motivate her to change some of that behavior contribute to the optimum development of the person supervised.

Administrators and their staffs can also profit from submitting to systematic observation of their behavior. It is unfortunate that the most significant parts of staff meetings occur in the corridors on the way *out* of the meeting. There is almost always something about the behavior of the administrator chairing the meeting that makes staff members reluctant to say what is on their minds. So the suggestions for improving operation and the gripes about perceptions of unfairness are communicated to peers, without ever reaching those who have the power to make changes. Not only, then, does the organization suffer from loss of important information, but those people who do the everyday work that keeps the organization going, are deprived of their feelings of pride, accomplishment, and great satisfaction that comes from having your ideas and feelings recognized as being important. Those administrators who really want staff input would find useful the information on an observation record to help them keep their behavior from interfering with their own objective.

Implications for the health field

There seems to be no reason why instruments for systematic observation cannot be used for similar objectives in the health field. In observing the interaction between health personnel and patients, nurses, aides, and even physicians could become more aware of their own behavior. They can become aware of the discrepancies between what they think their behavior is, and what they are actually doing. Above all, the person in any relationship who has less power and, consequently, less control over the development of the relationship, will be offered more opportunity to assume some measure of control. It is only through sharing control in an interactive situation that all the participants are left free to contribute everything they can and to continue unhampered the lifelong process of self-realization.

Just as in the field of education, observational techniques used in health care would be helpful in providing feedback to the one observed in order to raise the level of her awareness of her behavior. The practitioner could thus examine the observable consequences of her behavior and perhaps change her behavior so that the person with whom she is interacting is free to respond with his own feelings and needs. The comparison between education and nursing can very often be a one-to-one, point-by-point comparison, with the needs in education emerging as almost identical with the needs in nursing. In fact, nurses often say that a major aspect of their professional functioning is teaching.

Consider the matter of asking questions. The doctor who asks the patient, "How do you feel today?" immediately (1) continues reading the chart in his hand; (2) proceeds to prod and poke, sometimes asking specific questions related to the area under the prod, giving time to the patient for a quick yes, no, or grunt; (3) generally hears the answers to his questions from the nurse in attendance; (4) gives a direction or two to the nurse; (5) may or may not say a word of farewell to the patient before he disappears. The answer to the original question, "How do you feel today?" is largely *deduced* from other data—*not* from a specific answer by the patient. The significant aspects of the patient's response—including an opportunity to express his anxiety, fear, or anger; a purely subjective evaluation of his physical condition (so that efforts might be made to administer appropriate reassurances or other treatment); and an opportunity to ask for the kind of help he feels he needs—are inhibited by the physician's behavior. If asked about his behavior, the doctor would probably insist, in all honesty, that he most certainly does ask the patient questions and give him a chance to answer. However, if he were able to see a graphic representation of his behavior on an observation record, he would almost be compelled to see his behavior more realistically.

Similarly, the nurse who insists that she accepts the feelings of her patients, no matter what those feelings are, may be chagrined to see on the observation record that she accepts the feelings only of certain patients and not of others. She may deny the feelings of the patient who knows he is dying, by bombarding him with inappropriate attempts at gaiety and lightheartedness. She may be hostile to the woman who attempted with disastrous results to abort her own pregnancy. Her tight, disapproving lips may make it clear to the young man who attempted suicide that his feelings of terror and anger had better be kept to himself.

Ultimately, the nurse, like the teacher, must strive to help the people in her charge make the most of the situation in which they find themselves. The patient must learn some things about his condition and how to contribute to a certain measure of health and comfort for himself; he must maintain his image of himself as a worthwhile human being, in spite of what illness has done to him; he must be able to give and take freely in interactive situations with health personnel, members of his family, friends, and other patients.

The patient who needs to talk about his imminent death is not helped by the nurse who always includes a third party in her interactions with the patient. (A conversation with three people substantially reduces the possibility that any "dangerous" topic will be broached; it is not easy to confide in two people at once.) The man who needs to cry about his condition is not free to do so in the presence of a nurse who obviously expects of him the stoical behavior of her stereotypic male.

The interrelationships between nurses and their supervisors and administrators and their staffs also run parallel to similar relationships in the school setting. The student nurse is well aware of the trauma she experiences as she moves from one supervisor to another and from one service to another. It offers some comfort to know that most of her classmates are also suffering from the supervisor in obstetrics who always makes you feel inferior, or the one in medical-surgical who scares you so much that you invariably make mistakes. If such supervisors could see the objective record of their specific behaviors, they might choose to change those behaviors; thus students could have more productive relationships with the people who are teaching them.

It might be of particular interest to health personnel to have someone chart individual behaviors during a health team meeting. Of course, a record of observation should be shared *only* with the person observed. It is not to be used as the basis for general discussion—or gossip. The observed person is the one who must use the information and make a decision about whether or not to change his behavior. His behavior should *never* be recorded without his knowledge and consent.

The administrator who consents to have his behavior observed and recorded during a meeting may be in for some surprises. He may discover that, when he speaks, he looks only at the higher-echelon personnel and never at any of the other people around the table. (And he is so fond of saying that his office door is always open to everyone!) He may realize that the only question he ever asks is, "Is that clear to everyone?" (But he never waits for an answer even to that one!) He may be amazed to learn that he speaks for eighty percent of the total meeting time. (And he thought he conducted a democratic meeting!)

Generally, these are the reasons why the real agenda of a meeting usually goes on after the chairman adjourns. That's why so much of administration is just an unproductive spinning of wheels. That's why the level of efficient functioning in our society is so low. Policemen knew years ago that patroling the streets on foot was more likely to prevent crime than riding around in cars; police administrators are just now finding this out. Children have known all their lives that the things that are really important to them go on outside the classroom; teachers are just beginning to realize this. Dying patients have apparently always been aware of the fact that they were dying; nurses are just beginning to realize that their silence does not deceive the patient.

It is exciting to consider the possible effect of the widespread use of systematic observation in health care. Think of the nurse who believes he has overcome his reluctance to interact with dying patients. The observation feedback makes it clear that he consistently maintains a greater distance between himself and a dying patient than he does between himself and a patient who is expected to recover. He would, at the very least, be surprised at what the observation has revealed. He might go on to reexamine his feelings about dying patients. At the same time, he might make a conscious effort to shorten the distance between himself and each dying patient he talks with. The result may be improved communication as the patient perceives the growing proximity between himself and the nurse as evidence of affection and concern.

The nurse who is intellectually committed to the idea that patients have the right to honest answers to their questions may learn that her behavior actually discourages patients from asking questions, and thus saves her from the necessity of giving any answers. Her way of suppressing questions is to keep up a constant barrage of chatter while caring for the patient. The observation record makes it graphically clear that, although she spends much time with the patient and gives him excellent physical care, she permits no silence during her entire time at the bedside.

One doctor observed denied that she ever ordered patients around. However, in one six-minute session with a patient, she had given eight orders; the patient had time to respond to each with only a nod or a vague grunt of compliance. Following are her recorded orders:

> "We'll keep the catheter in; it saves the trouble of checking the urinal so often." (Technically, the patient could have managed without the catheter. But the aides had to check urine output more often if the urinal was used.)

"Better keep the flowers off the bed table; I almost knocked them over."

"Don't keep lying down all the time. It's better for you to sit up most of the time."

"I'm going to tell the nurse to limit your visiting time to one hour a day."

(In answer to a request transmitted by the nurse) "No wine in the hospital. It would set a bad precedent."

"I want you to eat everything on your tray."

"When your visitors come, let them do the talking; you just listen."

"Wear the hospital gown, not your own."

Conceivably, the medical orders were justified on the grounds that the patient's physical comfort was contingent upon compliance. But on what grounds could the other orders be justified, even those medical ones that really did not affect the patient's condition? Although the doctor immediately reacted to the feedback by trying to give acceptable reasons for the non-medical orders, she finally laughed at herself and admitted that she did sound fairly "bossy." Eventually, she conceded that she could give more complete explanations for her orders, so that the patient might better understand the reasons for them. (Not much of a concession, but progress is noted!)

chapter sixteen

———◆◀◉▶◆———

Instruments for
Observation

The process of recording and feedback

Though observation data are useful in all aspects of nursing, we are most concerned in the book with the observation of interaction between nurses and dying patients. Using the following simple instrument as a model, similar instruments may be developed that are more appropriate for observing relationships between supervisors and students, for example, or between nurses and patients who are expected to recover.

One of the objections to the use of an observational instrument while a patient is being treated might be the necessity for the observer to stand to one side and write while the nurse and the patient are interacting. Although this can conceivably detract somewhat from the intimacy and comfort of the situation, both patient and nurse may quickly forget—as they become absorbed in each other—that someone is recording their behavior. The patient will probably accept the explanation that this is a part of the training process. Patients in a teaching hospital generally tolerate well the inconveniences that accompany being cared for by students; therefore, observation by a third party will probably be accepted.

The person who is being observed, however, may find it a little more difficult. It is not easy to risk yourself to the critical analysis of your peers—nor even of your instructors, despite the practice we have all had in submitting our behavior to teacher evaluation. There should be, of course, a certain level of trust in the relationship, perhaps trust that has developed in the course of sharing feelings and ideas about death. If you can trust the observer not to condemn or ridicule behavior or to evaluate it in any way, but merely to *record* it, the observation process can be very fruitful.

The logical step after recording is to examine the behavior in terms of the likely consequences. The observed person can then make a decision about how to modify his own behavior so that he may obtain the desired results.

Sometimes, working as a group can help in the utilization of recorded observational data. However, this must be done in such a way that individuals are not exposed against their wills to the critical evaluation of the whole group. One way to use the data is to have one person collect all the observational records (from which the names of the observed have been deleted) and collate the behaviors on a single chart. The group can then use the chart as a basis for discussion. If, in the discussion, it becomes clear that there are differences in the values held, and thus differences in the desired results, the group may continue their study of values— defining, examining, and clarifying the various points of view. Individuals may decide to identify themselves as using a particular behavior and may even ask for assistance in changing their behavior. Obviously, these people trust their peers to be helpful and constructive in their responses.

The purpose of the observation instrument is merely to aid in recording behavior. What to do with that record is an individual's own decision. He may study it in private or discuss it in his group or tear it up in frustration and disgust.

The procedure of observation

1. Devise a list of behaviors to observe. The list may be supplemented as your experience with observation makes you more aware of other significant behaviors.
2. Pair up with another nurse.
3. One nurse should observe the other during a ten-minute period with a patient.
4. As you observe, put an "X" mark next to the behavior each time it is used.
5. After the observation, on a chart like the one pictured on page 174, put an X in the appropriate box for each X on the list. Where the X's cluster with the greatest frequency will indicate the general nature of your behavior with a patient: your readiness to listen, your

empathy, your sympathy, your neutrality, your avoidance, your fear. Where the X's cluster above the neutral box, your behavior encourages the patient to express his needs. The X's below the neutral box indicate that your behavior communicates to the patient that you want him to keep his needs to himself. The frequency with which the X's appear shows how often you used one or the other kind of behavior during the observation period.

6. Repeat this process with a patient in another condition. This time make O's on the list and on the chart. Now you can compare the two sets of marks to determine if your behavior with patients in different conditions varies, and in what areas, if any, that difference is apparent.

The observer should be careful to remain silent and not distract either the patient or the nurse being observed. Probably the best position for observing is a few inches to the right of the foot of the bed, facing the left corner of the head of the bed. Thus positioned, the observer has visual access to any point around the bed to which the nurse moves. At the same time, he is not in her way as she moves freely.

The nurse should, at all times during the ten-minute observation period, try to behave as if the observer were not there. She is not to say, "excuse me" as she goes past him, or include him in her conversation with the patient, or ask his assistance with anything.

It is a good idea to say to the patient at the outset—without elaboration or apology—"Mr. John's is observing me today. Do you mind if he just stands there and watches me?" Should the patient, by some remote chance, indicate any objection to this observation, then it must be abandoned. It is unlikely, however, that many patients would object.

The behaviors to observe

The list of behaviors below is arranged so that those behaviors which generally encourage the patient to be open about his needs come first. Proceeding down the list, the behaviors become less and less encouraging, until those behaviors are reached that actually seem to communicate to the patient that any open expression of his needs is neither expected nor wanted. Throughout the list, different clusters of behaviors indicate different motivations. This list was used for observing two ten-minute intervals so it does contain marks. The X marks record the behavior of a nurse and a patient; the O marks record the behavior of the same nurse with another patient.

Encouraging Patient's Expression of Needs

R **E** **A** **D** **I** **N** **E** **S** **S** **T** **O** **L** **I** **S** **T** **E** **N**	1. Sits down at bedside. 2. Sits for ten minutes.	
	3. Comes close to the patient without doing medical-technical things.	
	4. Asks, "Is there a question you'd like to ask me?"	X
	5. Invites the patient to ask questions.	
	6. Asks, "Is there something you would like to talk about?"	
	7. Asks, "How do you feel about being in the hospital?"	
	8. Asks, "How do you feel about the nurses here?"	
	9. Asks, "How do you feel about the doctors here?"	
	10. Asks, "How do you feel about the aides here?"	X
	11. Waits at least six seconds for the patient to respond to an invitation to speak.	
	12. Says, "Tell me more about how you feel."	X
	13. Accepts what the patient says.	X
	14. Says, "I've heard from other people that they feel that way when they come into the hospital."	
	15. Responds by building on what the patient said.	
E **M** **P** **A** **T** **H** **Y**	16. Looks at patient's face when she talks, nodding and murmuring understanding.	X
	17. Says, "Yes, I know. Something like that happened to me."	X
	18. Talks about death.	
	19. Talks about the patient's family.	
S **Y** **M** **P** **A** **T** **H** **Y**	20. Expresses sadness to match patient's sadness.	
	21. Expresses anger to match patient's anger.	
	22. Says, "I'm so sorry you have pain."	
	23. Says, "I'm so sorry I can't change things for you."	
	24. Cries when the patient cries.	

Neutral Behaviors That Are Part of Nurse's Responsibility

25. Works efficiently, doing what must be done for the patient's physical comfort.	X O
26. Routine directions. (Observer: make a mark for each direction.)	XXXXX XXX XX OCO

Discouraging Patient's Expression of Needs

A
V
O
I
D
A
N
C
E

27. Does not stop work even for a moment when patient is talking.	X O
28. Initiates talk only with casual pleasantry.	O
29. Responds to patient's casual talk with similar talk.	O

F
E
A
R

30. Does not talk to the patient except to give routine directions.	
31. Talks zestfully about the weather or view.	O
32. Acts brisk and "healthy," the kind of behavior that makes one say, "He's full of life!"	O
33. Asks a question and does not wait for an answer.	X
34. Keeps up a steady stream of small talk.	O
35. Comes in for a quick, "Anything you need?" and goes out again.	
36. Does not come close to patient except for specific nursing behaviors.	O
37. Stays with patient for less than five minutes.	O
38. Does not respond when the patient says something.	O
39. Leaves without responding when the patient says something.	X

Charting the behavior

On page 174 is a chart giving a graphic presentation of the behaviors of one nurse in her interaction with two patients. The marks next to the behaviors on the preceding list have been written in the appropriate spaces on the chart. Thus, behavior #4, which was observed one time in the ten-minute observation, is put on the chart in the *Readiness to Listen* space. Behavior #27 is put on the chart in the *Avoidance* space. etc.

When all the behaviors were charted in this way, the nurse was able to see at a glance just what she had been doing.

Discussion

On this chart, the X's give a picture of the nurse's interaction with a patient recovering from minor surgery. The O's present the nurse's interaction with a patient dying of cancer. Of course, the differences do not always emerge so clearly, but here we can see that even the neutral behaviors are substantially reduced during interaction with the dying patient. There is no behavior that indicates readiness to listen to either the dying patient or the recovering one. However, there is strong evidence of avoidance and fear of the dying patient.

This particular nurse readily admitted the accuracy of the picture to her observer, but insisted that it was the behavior of the patient that caused her reactions and that she would not behave in the same way with every dying patient. The observer did not argue with her, but they agreed to continue the observation to see if a consistent pattern of behavior became apparent. It was not very long before this nurse discovered that she *did* treat dying patients differently from the way she treated patients who were expected to recover. By that time, other people in her group were beginning to admit the same thing about themselves. Therefore, her discovery was not quite so disturbing and depressing as it might have been if she thought she was different from everyone else— "unprofessional," perhaps. The energy in the group, then, rather than being used in defensive efforts was used to help each other change behavior.

Other suggestions for observation

There are other, simpler ways to make a systematic observation by concentrating on a single behavior. For your own information, you may count the number of visits staff members make to dying patients and compare them with the number of visits made to patients who are expected to recover. If you see a pattern emerge—fewer visits overall to dying patients, fewer *casual* visits to dying patients—you may learn something about how dealing with death is being managed in your institu-

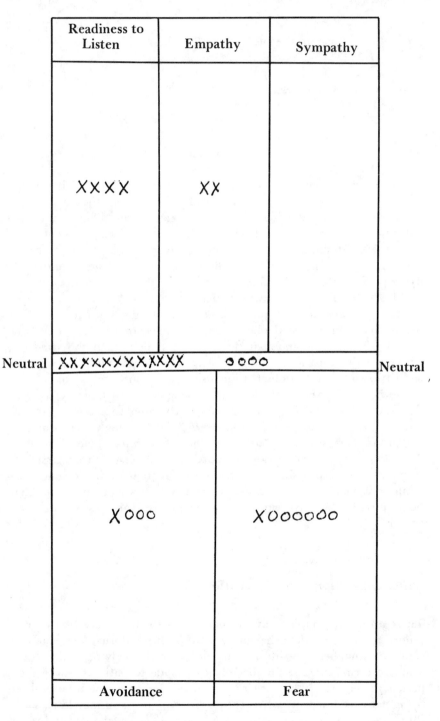

tion. Compare this pattern to your own pattern of visitation. Is there a difference in the number and kind of your visits to a patient before a diagnosis of terminal illness and after such a diagnosis?

If you want to engage in a somewhat more specific observation of your colleagues, count the number of visits to a terminally ill patient during each of the stages of dying—denial, anger, bargaining, acceptance. Does a pattern emerge here? Is there a stage during which visits decrease significantly? Is there a stage during which there are no social or casual visits—but visits only to provide essential medical and nursing treatment?

If you wish to discuss the tabulated results of your observation in a class or a staff meeting, the anonymity of the observed individuals should be respected. Actually, the behaviors of individuals are not immediately at issue here. It seems more important to discover what the general approach to dying patients is in a hospital, so that there may be general discussion of policy and philosophy. Perhaps it is only after such a general observation and discussion that staff members can begin to think about their own behaviors with regard to making some changes.

Situations for simulated observation

It would be inconsistent with the plan of this book to expect either students or practioners to submit themselves to observation procedures in a real setting without some opportunity to improve the specific skills needed and to achieve some measure of comfort with the whole process. Consequently, the observation procedure should first be tried a number of times in simulated situations before it is tried at the bedside of a real patient.

Any of the cases throughout the book may be used for practice. In addition, the descriptions of situations beginning on page 176 may also be useful. For each situation follow the procedure for observation exactly as described. However, in simulation, the rest of the class may also tabulate the behavior while the observer and the nurse are role playing the scene. Afterwards, the observation records may be compared and some of the difficulties of observation discussed. The reasons for differences among observers and the feelings of the people observed, etc., should also be considered.

This kind of group observation should *never* be attempted in a real situation. One observer is enough for any nurse or patient! More than one observer would undoubtedly change the nature of the relationship between the nurse and the patient and thus reveal a pattern that is not typical of what happens between nurse and patient. Feedback of such atypical behavior would not be useful to the nurse who is trying to analyze and modify her own behavior.

The situations that follow are variations on a single theme. The characters in each are the same people. What changes in each case are the prognosis, the patient's knowledge of her own death, and the patient's dying trajectory. Because the characters are the same, a person playing a character may have a tendency to repeat his behaviors out of habit. Therefore, an individual should role play the nurse in only one situation during a session.

If a group observation is made, the differences in individual data may be discussed. A comparison of the methods of different role-players should also be made.

An alternative way of using the situations is to eliminate all references in the story to the key point. For example, in Situation #2, leave out the following sentences: "The original illness is consequently complicated by this new development and the medical consensus is that Ms. S. is terminal; she is not expected to live more than one month. No one has told her this." Before you start the observation session, send the "nurse" out of the room, and give everyone else the information in these two sentences. Then observe the nurse's behavior.

After ten minutes, tell the "nurse" the information in those sentences and continue your observation of her behavior, using another colored pencil.

Still another approach is to use two or more of the situations at one time. Put "patient #1" in one bed and in an adjacent bed "patient #2." The "nurse" is to know only that both patients are the same, as the accounts reveal. What the "nurse" does not know—and what the observers do know—is that the first "patient" is expected to die in one month. The "nurse" spends ten minutes with the first "patient" while the observers record behavior. Then she spends ten minutes with the second "patient," while the observers record behavior with another colored pencil. Afterwards, the "nurse" can compare her behavior with each "patient."

Situation #1

Ms. S. is a white, Jewish woman of forty-four, married, and the mother of three teen-age children. She has just had major surgery to correct previous surgery. The operation has apparently not corrected the condition, and the patient is in great discomfort, forced to lie face down all the time. She does so with no complaining, for the most part suffering the discomfort in silence. In conversations with the staff, she talks about her family and the community volunteer work that was so much a part of her life.

Mr. G., the nurse assigned to her during the day, comes in.

Situation #2

Ms. S. is a white, Jewish woman of forty-four, married, and the mother of three teen-age children. She has just had major surgery to correct previous surgery. The operation has apparently not corrected the condition, and the patient is in great discomfort, forced to lie face down all the time. The original illness is complicated by this new development and the medical consensus is that Ms. S. is terminally ill. She is not expected to live more than one month. No one has told her this.

For the most part, Ms. S. suffers in silence. In conversations with the staff, she talks about her family and the community volunteer work that was so much a part of her life.

Mr. G., the nurse assigned to her during the day, comes in.

Situation #3

Ms. S. is a white, Jewish woman of forty-four, married, and the mother of three teen-age children. She has just had major surgery to correct previous surgery. The operation has apparently not corrected the condition, and the patient is in great discomfort, forced to lie face down all the time. She does so with no complaining, for the most part suffering the discomfort in silence. In conversations with the staff, she talks about her family and the community volunteer work that was so much a part of her life.

Mr. G., the nurse assigned to her during the day, comes in. Mr. G. has had some experience with this condition. He had a patient who had been through exactly the same thing and had died unexpectedly one week after the last surgery. As far as he knows, Ms. S.'s prognosis is favorable—there is no expectation that she will die. But Mr. G. can't help remembering his other patient.

Situation #4

Ms. S. is a white, Jewish woman of forty-five, married, and the mother of three teen-age children. She has just had major surgery to correct previous surgery. The operation has apparently not corrected the condition, and the patient is in great discomfort, forced to lie face down all the time. In addition, Ms. S. knows that the original illness cannot be arrested, and that she has no more than a year to live.

For the most part Ms. S. does not complain. In conversations with the staff, she talks about her family and the community volunteer work that was so much a part of her life.

Mr. G., the nurse assigned to her during the day, comes in.

section seven

---◄◆►---

Helping the Professional

chapter seventeen

———❖———

Reducing the Feeling
of Isolation

The need for help

In learning to help the dying patient and his family, we must be careful
not to overlook the fact that the nurse also needs help. If the *inevitability*
of our own deaths is not so easy to deal with, neither is the *possibility* that
we may one day have the illness we happen to be treating. And each dying
patient becomes a reminder that we, too, one day will be dying.

Just as family and friends of the patient suffer from loss and the feelings
surrounding loss, so the nurse also may suffer bereavement. The question
is, "Who helps the nurse?" No general hospital currently provides a per-
manent structure or procedure for helping its staff cope productively with
the effects of interacting with dying people. Nor are staff personnel given
even casual institutional help for working through their feelings and recovering from the death of a patient. Generally, the effort is made to establish a norm of stoicism and something called "professionalism," which
seems to mean little more than just hiding feelings.

One of the problems that doctors and nurses have when faced with the
social-psychological needs of dying people, is that they themselves often
do not have the psychological resources for fulfilling those needs. This is
especially true of personnel in specialties where a high percentage of
patients are suffering from terminal illness. It becomes an emotional burden for the doctor or nurse to establish open, empathic communication
with every such patient—too much grief, too much sadness, too great a
sense of futility and failure.

Some people in the field have suggested that there be specialists—thanatologists, if you will—who take on the task of helping patients to die. Maybe this is an answer, but it seems to be a little too pat. We have a tendency to create a specialty whenever we become aware of a lack in professional functioning. However, it might be wise to consider that nurses, physicians, and aides must interact with the dying person day after day, from minute to minute. While handling a patient's medical treatment, they cannot ignore the dying, the awareness of dying, the feelings about dying. The dying person cannot be held in reserve for the visit and the expert ministrations of the thanatologist, so that other health personnel are freed from the anxieties of interacting with a person who is dying.

Characteristically, however, it is those in need who will have to take the initiative for fulfilling their own needs. Those who feel the pain and the urgency are the ones who are most likely to take measures to reduce the pain. The helpers themselves must marshal their resources and systematically help each other whenever needed.

Such help depends on a heightened awareness of the need, and on the development of helping skills. Each nurse is well aware that he has strong responsive feelings when he treats a dying patient, and that he mourns when the patient dies. His mourning may be rigidly controlled and hidden from everyone else. He may believe that there is something unprofessional or even weak about having such feelings. So, when we speak of awareness of need in helping the professional, we must be concerned specifically with seeing through the sometimes desperate attempts to hide the need. Probably the most important way to become aware of this need is to create a working atmosphere that encourages individuals to admit that they do need help, and that such an admission is no reflection on their professional competency. As time goes on and one person after another profits from the help, the norm of responding to death and dying will change, and the stereotype of the unemotional nurse will be destroyed. Most significantly, nurses will no longer have to bear the burden of their feelings alone.

The development of helping skills is probably much more easily done than changing the professional norm of expressing feelings. In the safety of the classroom one can hopefully sharpen his sensitivity to an individual's specific need and develop a repertory of behaviors on which to draw once the need is identified. The following exercise contributes to both of these.

Practicing helping

List on a chart or the chalkboard the following *categories* of help that might be needed by a nurse who is treating a dying patient, or whose patient has just died. Add other categories if you wish, if the list seems incomplete.

Categories of Help

1. Non-verbal	2. Verbal	3. Activities	4. Just leave him alone

bodily contact
listening
kinesthetic
  response with-
  out contact
  (body
  language)
	explanations
	reassurances
	advice
		entertainment
		help with the
		  dying patient
		  and/or his
		  family
		accompany to
		  eating,
		  walking, etc.	

Break up into groups of eight or nine people. Each person should have a turn at playing the role of the nurse in the following story. One person should read the story aloud, while the rest listen and try to put themselves in the nurse's place.

Jim Gordon is an experienced and competent nurse, assigned to the medical-surgical floor of City Hospital. In the past three weeks, three of his patients have died. Two of them had been in the hospital periodically for months. The third had been admitted a week ago and had died very quickly. He had come to know each patient in a special way and had liked them all.

One of them, Mr. Tesconi, was an old man. He had a loving family of children and grandchildren. He even had three great-grandchildren, of whom he was very proud. The family had rallied around him when he became ill, and, though they knew he was going to die, they had behaved as if he had another lifetime ahead of him. They brought him food and gifts from home; there was always someone at his bedside; they assisted the staff in nursing him, and in every way—except talking about dying—they made his last weeks much like the rest of his life had been.

Jim Gordon had developed great affection for the old man and his family. They included the nurse in the warmth of the family as if he were one of them. During difficult times, when the fact of death could not be put aside, it was Jim in whom they confided. There were long periods of time when Jim sat with his patient in the quiet hours of the night, just holding his hand, saying nothing.

The second patient was a young mother of two small children. For a long time after she learned she was dying, she was furiously angry. She lashed out at everyone—family, friends, the staff—and especially at the nurse who cared for her during the day. For weeks, Jim absorbed all the anger, responding with vague words of reassurance and administering the medical procedures as gently as he could. Sometimes he would spare a few minutes to sit quietly and listen to her words of anger that barely hid the despair and terror underneath.

Finally, Ms. Green began to talk about her children and her husband, crying at the thought of leaving them, worrying about who would care for them with the kind of devotion she wanted them to have. At first, it was only Jim that she could take into her confidence, sharing the same anxieties with him over and over again. Gradually, he was able to draw her husband into these confidences, but Ms. Green, until she died, was never willing to relinquish her relationship with Jim.

The third patient was Bob Johnson, a man about Jim's age. He appeared to be healthy and had almost no symptoms. It was hard to believe that the small lump on his knee resulted in a diagnosis of cancer that had metastasized extensively, and the decision that nothing more could be done for him. Apparently, the patient, too, could not believe that he would soon die. He talked to Jim about his plans for the future and laughed a lot with his friends who came to visit him.

It was only at night, when the floor was quiet, that he would ask Jim to sit with him for a while. It was at these times that he would ask Jim if he ever thought about dying. Until the patient died one morning, he continually oscillated between awareness that he was going to die and apparent confidence that he had only a minor illness.

Now that each listener has heard what Jim Gordon has experienced in the past three months, he must have some idea of how Jim feels. One person should *be* Jim Gordon for a while, remembering Mr. Tesconi, Ms. Green, and Bob Johnson.

Anyone in the group may ask the nurse questions if he feels that additional information will be useful in his attempts to help. The nurse may respond with information about himself, his patients, the nature of the work he has been doing, the experiences he has been having, his feelings—anything he thinks will help his colleagues help him.

One at a time, the rest of the group can say or do something that he thinks will help Jim. After each attempt to help, let "Jim" say what this did for him: if it really did help, and how; if it made him feel worse; if the attempt had no meaning.

Let each person in the group try to "help" until Jim is able to say that a particular attempt was what he needed. Then, someone else can be Jim, and the same procedure followed.

After the exercise is completed, the group might discuss their ideas about helping. Have you changed some of the ideas you started with? Do you remember the Golden Rule: Do unto others as you would have them do unto you? Well, have you discovered that what *you* might need in such a situation is not necessarily what someone else needs? Maybe the best thing you can do with the Golden Rule is substitute the Judaic version: Do not do unto others what you would not have others do unto you. Or maybe you ought to scrap *all* maxims and concentrate on the real person in front of you and what he is trying to communicate to you. Have you found some ways of determining what another person under stress needs from you? Do you agree with the generalization that men don't need as much help in dealing with grief as women do? Why or why not? (Another time, you might try the exercise with a woman as the nurse in the story, and see if the nature of the proffered help changes.)

Organizing to help

If you conclude that the nurse who must deal with death and dying can find the help of colleagues useful, perhaps you might consider the possibility of organizing for such help. Whether you are at this point in time working on your pre-service or your in-service education, it is not impossible to undertake such organization. At first, this idea may sound completely impractical. Actually, however, organization does not need to be a complicated undertaking. Here are several guidelines that may help you refrain from attempting more than you can handle:

1) Do not feel that you need everyone, or even a majority of your colleagues, committed to your organization. Just one or two other likeminded people should be enough of an "organization."

2) The key to success is not complexity of structure, large blocks of free time, or even administrative approval. The simple model of interpersonal interaction needs no trappings of a large organization, nor can it be easily interdicted by arbitrary authority.

3) The success of your helping organization will depend on the consistency of the help you provide for each other. Whatever approach you decide to use, you must use it every time, including everyone who is experiencing the dying or death of a fellow human being. All of you must begin to *expect* help to be forthcoming when it is needed. This expectation is the essence of structure. When people begin to look to each other for help as a matter of course, and are not disappointed, the organization is truly operating. Perhaps you and some of your colleagues—in your class, in your study group, or on your floor—could set up such a simple structure designed for mutual aid. It could go into action whenever someone called for help, or simply seemed to need it. Even if only one person in the group spotted a clue that indicated need, he could alert the rest of the people and set the helping mechanism in motion.

Perhaps part of such a plan should be to meet regularly, just to *ask* if anyone needs help. Other people may join the group if the members make it abundantly clear that they are not an exclusive group, that they speak freely about their objectives, and that they want the commitment and involvement to spread. If they continue to function regularly and openly—even if, for a long time, the functioning means only sitting together once or twice a week and talking openly about their interest—direct proselytizing will probably not be necessary. The need for such an organization is so great that it must inevitably draw people to it.

If something practical is not done to help nurses handle their emotions about dying patients, then the sad coverups will continue. Recently, a patient who was particularly impressed with the pleasant smile and skillful hands of a nurse expressed the hope that he would see her on the following day. The nurse explained to him that the hospital's policy was to rotate nurses, so that no one nurse would become too involved with any one patient. Evidently, this policy had been devised to reduce the possibility that a nurse would develop any strong feelings about a patient. By implication, the policy said that should a nurse in spite of avoidance still feel strongly about a patient, the fault was her own: the organization provided a mechanism for avoidance. Without organizational sanction, whatever feelings the nurse had were inappropriate and, therefore, better kept to herself.

Perhaps if nurses themselves engaged in a helping plan such as the one described in this book, some of the residual fear of involvement that is so much a part of the medical profession could be eliminated. Naturally, no nurse will feel the same pleasure in every patient's company, nor will he grieve the same for every dying patient. But pleasure and pain are essential factors in human relationships. The person who denies or suppresses his feelings does not communicate scientific objectivity; he communicates *that he does not care.* There is no greater emotional communication than that!

To take over major control of another person's body, to make life and death decisions for him *is* involvement. There is no way to avoid involvement with patients; it is a function of medical care. But the responsibilities that go along with involvement need not be borne by individuals alone. The professional group or the social group should be a part of the involvement process. When involvement in the dying of a patient proves too difficult for one person, the group, recognizing the inevitable involvement of us all in the process of dying, can take on some of the responsibility for sharing the burden.

Lest someone persist in saying, "All of this is idealistic. It will never work in the practical everyday work world," may I suggest that it merely is the logical extension of what is done on the job every day? Who would suggest that increasing nursing personnel as the patient population increases is "idealistic"? And don't we increase the number of dressings as the number of surgical procedures increase? Why not, then, increase the quantity of emotional support as the emotion increases in a particular situation?

Making contact with the world

When we experience the death of someone close to us—whether it is a member of our family, or a patient for whom we have learned to care deeply—we are often beset with feelings of anger, despair, and guilt that seem almost overwhelming. It seems as if no one has ever felt this way, that these feelings are uniquely attributable to all the ways we failed in our relationship with the dead person, everything we are that invited punishment and retribution from the fates.

It is possible to get some relief from these feelings by becoming aware of their universality, by discovering that people throughout the ages have felt the same and have struggled—in their grief and anguish—to understand the meaning of life and death.

When we find ourselves unable to put our feelings into words, the poet may be able to help us. When we have experiences that make us feel isolated, alone, apart from the rest of humankind, we may turn to the novelist for evidence that we are not alone. It is sometimes easier to be able to say, "Yes, that's exactly what I mean!" than to communicate our meaning in our own words.

Here are a few observations of writers who, perhaps, have been able to put into words what all of us feel at one time or another. If they scratch open an old wound and make you cry for someone long gone, let the tears come. "Deposits of unfinished grief reside in more American hearts than I ever realized" (Kavanaugh).

Chih Ming, fourteen hundred years ago, cried

> Unreal
> Unreal are both creation
> And destruction,
> And man's body
> Is delusion and a dream.[1]

unwilling to believe that the real self could be so fragile, could perish so quickly.

Conrad, thirteen centuries later bemoaned the fact that

> There is never time to say our last word—the last word of our love, of our desire, faith, remorse, submission, revolt.[2]

---

[1] "Facing Death," trans. by Henry H. Hart, in *World Literature*, Christy & Wells, Eds, American Book Co., New York, N.Y., p. 168.

[2] "Lord Jim," in *The Portable Conrad*, Morton Dauwen Zabel, Ed., The Viking Press, New York, N.Y., p. 721.

Shelley denied death altogether:

> Peace, peace! he is not dead, he doth not sleep—
> He hath awakened from the dream of life—

And in the same breath, he begged the dead to return and leave him
with one more memory:

> Stay yet awhile! speak to me once again;
> Kiss me, so long but as a kiss may live;
> And in my heartless breast and burning brain
> That word, that kiss, shall all thoughts else survive,
> With food of saddest memory kept alive,
> Now thou art dead, as if it were a part
> Of thee, my Adonais! [1]

Wordsworth mourned a dead child and at the same time saw him well
out of the troubles of life:

> For *he* is safe, a quiet bed
> Hath early found among the dead,
> Harboured when none can be misled,
>   Wronged, or distrest;
> And surely here it may be said
>   that such are blest.[2]

Landor wondered of what use it was to have beauty and virtue and
grace, as long as death is inevitable, and cried unconsolably:

> Rose Aylmer, whom these wakeful eyes
>   May weep, but never see [3]

Whitman sang strongly of the universality of death and praised it as
he did all things in life:

> Come lovely and soothing death,
> Undulate round the world, serenely
>   arriving, arriving,
> In the day, in the night, to all, to each
> Sooner or later delicate death.
>   . . .
>   . . . praise! praise! praise!
> For the sure-enwinding arms of
>   cool-enfolding death.[4]

---

[1] "Adonais," *English Romantic Poems,* Stephen, Beck & Snow, Eds., American Book Co.,
New York, N.Y., pp. 497-506.
[2] "At the Grave of Burns," ibid., pp. 61-62.
[3] "Rose Aylmer," *World Literature,* op. cit., p. 733.
[4] "When Lilacs Last in the Boryard Bloomed," ibid., pp. 651-654.

Voltaire shrugged his shoulders, and accepted that the moment of death—like everything else in life—was predestined:

> Imbeciles say: "My doctor has saved my aunt from a mortal malady; he has made her life ten years longer than she ought to have lived." [1]

Sandburg comforted himself and wryly soothed his own fears:

> Death is a nurse mother with big arms: 'Twon't
> hurt you at all; it's your time now;
> you just need a long sleep, child; what have
> you had anyhow better than sleep? [2]

Alfred de Musset knew, as do contemporary psychologists, that the grieving would help to calm the anger and put the loss into the past, where it properly belonged:

> I will not dry these tear-drops: let
> them flow,
> And soothe a bitterness that yet might last,
> And o'er my waking eyelids throw
> The shadow of the past. [3]

And Wordsworth feared death in the midst of life—and at the height of love:

> What fond and wayward thoughts will slide
> Into a Lover's head!
> "O mercy!" to myself I cried,
> "If Lucy should be dead!" [4]

And yesterday, a young woman saw her mother die and she could not believe that the mother who was there one moment was no longer there the next. She denied death, felt guilty that she had not made good what was bad between them, then was grateful that the suffering was over— for both of them. She cried and cried until she was able to dry her eyes, look about her again, and see that death was the end for us all. Now, for the rest of her life, she will cry a little with every dying person, until the day when someone who cares will cry a little with her.

---

[1] "Selections; Destiny," in *The Portable Voltaire*, The Viking Press, op. cit., p. 105.
[2] "Death Snips Proud Men," reprinted from *Smoke and Steel* in *Selected Poems of Carl Sandburg*, Rebecca West, Ed., Harcourt, Brace & Co., New York, p. 186.
[3] "Souvenir," in *World Literature*, op. cit., pp. 647-650.
[4] "Strange Fits of Passion Have I Known," *English Romantic Poems*, op. cit., p. 28.

chapter eighteen

Confronting an Essential Conflict

The conflict defined

In many contemporary textbooks on the fundamentals of nursing care there is no mention of death or dying. Every discussion of treatment or interaction stops short of the dying patient. The inevitable inference that the reader must make is that a nurse is concerned with whether a person is sick or well; dying is apparently not one of the fundamentals. One book that does have a chapter on death and grief admits that "Effective performance in nursing care is usually oriented toward the patient's progress and health. . . . (Schwartz and Schwartz, *The Psychodynamics of Patient Care*).

Quint says frankly, "The death of a patient is in conflict with the primary life-saving goals of the hospital. . . . In general, dying patients do not provide the same satisfactions as do patients who recover." ("The Dying Patient: A Difficult Nursing Problem," *Nursing Clinics of North America*, December, 1967.)

Given the professional commitment to prolong life, the fact of a dying patient must cause anxiety for medical personnel. Even the medical opinion "there is nothing more we can do" states very clearly that when life can no longer be prolonged, our function in regard to that patient ceases. At this time do we shrug off our feeling of helplessness and failure by separating ourselves from the patient who is dying? Do we reject the sense of failure by rejecting the patient who is dying?

Perhaps it would be helpful if published definitions of nursing were more explicit about dying or death. Instead of including only the words illness and suffering, prevention and coping, we ought also to define nursing in terms of living and dying, so that the dying patient may never again be turned over to another service (religion? social work? thanatology?) while he is still living.

An Exercise in Values Clarification

| It is ridiculous to suppose that anyone could get any satisfaction out of treating a patient who shortly dies | | Treating a patient who shortly dies can be a very satisfying experience. |

Where do you stand on this continuum, at one extreme or the other, or somewhere in between? Put your mark on that point on the line where your feeling seems to fit, and write a brief description of your attitude concerning satisfaction in treating the dying patient.

Now, get together in small groups, making sure that the various attitudes in the group fall on a variety of points on the continuum, from one end to the other. Sit in a semicircle facing a chalkboard or chart paper and draw the continuum again, putting your marks in the same places on the continuum as you did before. Now you have a picture of how your small group is divided on this issue.

Before you begin to talk to each other, expand in writing the description of your attitude that you wrote when you first decided where you fell on the continuum. For example, if your description fell at the right end of the line, list some of the specific satisfactions that you might have from treating a dying patient. If your description fell at the left end of the continuum, list all the reasons why satisfaction in such a nursing situation is impossible. If you found that your point of view falls somewhere between the two ends of the continuum, perhaps you can list satisfactions in one column and blocks to satisfaction in the other, and so justify your being closer to one end of the line than the other.

In the semicircle, share your satisfactions and what you see as obstacles to satisfaction in treating a dying patient. As you participate in the discussion, add to your own list points that had not occurred to you and that you now want to accept as your own. On the other hand, if someone makes you see that what you thought would be a good part of the experience is really disgusting, you should cross out the point in your satisfactions column and add it to your dissatisfactions column.

As your perceptions of satisfaction and dissatisfaction are modified, you may need to move from your original spot on the continuum closer to one end or the other. Don't be afraid to change as often as you feel the need. At the end of the discussion you may even find that you need to think about this matter more—and have more experiences with people who are dying—before you can say for sure what your attitude is.

If you have difficulty in making up your mind re-examine your original reason for becoming a nurse. Did you want to help make sick people well again? Did you think about contributing to the relief of suffering? (Did relief of suffering mean the same to you as curing disease?) Were you interested in preventive medicine? If these are the objectives you had in mind when you decided to choose nursing as a vocation, can you see how death really blocks the achievement of your objectives? Obviously, each time a patient dies, you have failed in (1) making a sick person well again; (2) curing a disease; (3) preventing someone from being sick.

Does this seem to apply to you? Are you having trouble reconciling your need to cure with the inevitability of a patient's death? And since death *is* inevitable, can you see no way of getting some satisfaction from the experience while you are feeling frustration and disappointment?

Perhaps some of the other people in your group can help you recognize some possible satisfactions in interacting with a dying patient. At any rate, be assured that the inner conflict you are experiencing is understandable. As you add to your experiences in learning to interact with dying patients, you might continue to adjust your two columns and your spot on the continuum, until you feel you have resolved the conflict for yourself.

An Exercise in Identifying Differential Treatment

Break up into small groups, and give each group a number. All the odd-numbered groups should do the following exercise:

Directions for odd-numbered groups

On a sheet of paper write the heading, *Patient with Appendicitis.* Under it list all the things a nurse does *for* and *with* the patient who has been admitted to the hospital with a diagnosis of appendicitis. *Do not include in your list the necessary medical and surgical procedures.* Write down only those things that might be labeled psychological, social, personal, and human behaviors, and give some indication of how much time should be spent doing them. Don't forget to include topics of conversation, too. Take all of fifteen minutes to do this, so you may be sure that you are not putting down only those things that occur to you immediately, and leaving out some things that you have to "dig" for a little.

Directions for even-numbered groups

On a sheet of paper, write the heading, *Patient with Acute Lymphosarcoma*. Under it list all the things a nurse does *for* and *with* the patient who has been diagnosed as having acute lymphosarcoma. *Do not include in your list the necessary medical and surgical procedures.* Write down only those things that might be labeled psychological, social, personal, and human behaviors, and give some indication of how much time should be spent doing them. Don't forget to include topics of conversation, too. Take all of fifteen minutes to do this, so you may be sure that you are not putting down only those things that occur to you immediately, and leaving out some things that you have to "dig" for a little.

Directions for all groups

At the end of fifteen minutes, rearrange yourselves into larger groups, each made up of one odd-numbered and one even-numbered group. Each newly-formed group should compare the "Appendicitis" lists with the "Lymphosarcoma" lists.

Questions to Help in Your Comparisons

1. Are you finding some things in the "Appendicitis" lists that also appear every time on the "Lymphosarcoma" lists? Write these things on a chart or on the chalkboard. Head them *Common Behaviors*.
2. Are there some things in the "Appendicitis" lists that do *not* appear on the "Lymphosarcoma" lists? Write these things on a chart or on the chalkboard. Head them *Behaviors for Appendicitis*.
3. Are there some things in the "Lymphosarcoma" lists that do not appear on the "Appendicitis" lists? Head them *Behaviors for Lymphosarcoma*.
4. Do you see a pattern emerging in each list? For example, do the behaviors on the "Appendicitis" list generally require more time than the behaviors on the "Lymphosarcoma" list? How do you account for this?

   Are there fewer behaviors on the "Lymphosarcoma" list than on the "Appendicitis" list? How do you account for this?

Are the behaviors of the "Lymphosarcoma" list characterized by some aspects that make them essentially different from the behaviors on the "Appendicitis" list? For example, do the behaviors on the "Appendicitis" list generally require more touching of the patient than do the behaviors on the "Lymphosarcoma" list? Are the topics of conversation on the "Lymphosarcoma" list more general, less related to the patient's illness? Are they more determinedly "cheerful" topics?

5. Do you believe that there are essential differences in patient care, depending on whether the patient's prognosis is favorable or unfavorable? Or do you think that good patient care is the same—except for specific medical-surgical procedures—whether the patient is suffering from appendicitis or acute lymphosarcoma?

If you believe there must be differences, how do you justify that belief? Is your justification based on evidence that the dying patient really has different needs? (Do you know what the needs of dying patients are? Or are you basing your reasons on *your* needs and *your* feelings?)

An Exercise in Changing Behavior

Role play the following situation:

John Wyman is a thirty-eight-year-old man who has just been admitted to the hospital with a kidney infection. He is not in great discomfort. This is the fifth or sixth recurrence of the infection over a period of four years. He has taken his doctor's advice to enter the hospital and undergo intensive testing to find out what is causing his problem.

Mr. Wyman is a teacher. He is a good-looking, personable man, and the personnel who come into contact with him like him immediately. He has many friends who call him on the telephone. He has asked people not to visit him, since he is only in the hospital for an examination and should be back home and at work in a few days. Since he is not married and his parents are not living, his wishes have apparently been respected, and no one has come to visit.

Ellen Downs is a nursing student assigned to care for Mr. Wyman. She likes him, enjoys talking to him, and spends as much time with him as she possibly can.

This morning, he is sitting in a chair while she changes the linen on his bed. They are talking about the tests he underwent the previous day, and wondering what they revealed. Several times the subject of his work has come up, and he has expressed some concern about his students and the work they must complete before the end of the semester.

Pick up the role-playing at this point, continuing the conversation.

While Mr. Wyman and Ms. Downs talk, the rest of the class should take notes on what is happening. The following questions may serve as suggestions for note-taking. Do not limit your observations to these questions. Write down anything about the interaction that strikes you as significant.

1. What would you say is the mood of the conversation?
2. Do you have any indication of Mr. Wyman's feelings—about the tests, the possible prognosis, being in the hospital?
3. How does Ms. Downs seem to feel about Mr. Wyman? Does she seem generally to be comfortable with him, or do you detect some discomfort? If you detect discomfort, can you identify the source?

After a reasonable time of role-playing and observation, stop the action and put your notes aside.

Mr. Wyman and Ms. Downs are now talking to each other again. However, it is now the next day. Again Ms. Downs is straightening the room. Yesterday, both Ms. Downs and Mr. Wyman learned the results of the tests: he has carcinoma that has metastasized and he will not live long.

While Mr. Wyman and Ms. Downs are role playing, the rest of the class should take notes again, using the same questions as guidelines. After a reasonable time, stop the action.

The two people who played Mr. Wyman and Ms. Downs should join the rest of the class. The class should compare the results of their observations, and try to find similarities and differences between the first and second conversations. Mr. Wyman and Ms. Downs can make contributions when they feel it appropriate, indicating how the observers' interpretations compared with what they were feeling and trying to communicate.

Did you find marked differences between the two scenes? Could you conclude that knowledge of Mr. Wyman's imminent death resulted in clearly observable changes in mood, apparent feelings, and topics of conversation? Which scene was played for a longer period of time? To what do you attribute the difference in length of conversation?

Would anybody in the group like to take the opportunity to change the second scene, re-play it in another way? Perhaps Ms. Downs, after thinking it over, would like to stay with Mr. Wyman for a longer period of time. Perhaps Mr. Wyman would like to test out different ways of introducing the subject of his illness and impending death. Perhaps Ms. Downs would like to try out behavior that was not so obviously nervous.

Feel free to use this scene in any way you wish to practice skills, to get some clues to your own and others' feelings, or merely to say what you feel the need to say at this moment. Just remember, any mistakes you make in interaction during role-playing are easily correctable. Just go back and do it over again if you don't like the way you did it the first time. That's what makes role-playing so much safer than real life!

An Exercise in Developing Consistency Between Philosophy and Behavior

Here is the transcript of a conversation between two nurses concerning the treatment of a patient to whom both have been assigned. How would you change any part of the conversation to make it more consistent with your own philosophy of nursing?

NURSE A: Hi. You can leave now. I'll finish filing the charts.

NURSE B: Great! I'm really tired today.

NURSE A: Anything I ought to know?

NURSE B: Well, Mrs. Ganon has been having some pain. I think she's all right for the night, but if she isn't she may need a repeat of her medication.

NURSE A: How about Mrs. Barnes? Did you get her up today?

NURSE B: Yes! And you should have heard her complain! I think she'd be very happy to just lie in bed for several weeks and let everyone wait on her.

NURSE A: I can't say I blame her. This is a vacation for her from those six children!

NURSE B: Well, she was sorry to hear that she'll be out of here by to-morrow.

NURSE A: Anything else?

NURSE B: No. Nothing new on the others. Oh, uh, there's Mrs. Crandor, of course. Poor thing.

NURSE A: Um-m-m.

NURSE B: She needs a lot of reassurance. She's so depressed—so upset all the time.

NURSE A: Maybe increased medication would help. After all, there isn't much to be done except to make her as comfortable as possible.

NURSE B: I really ought to talk to her some more, but I just don't have the time.

NURSE A: Well, none of us do. Don't feel guilty; you do the best you can.

NURSE B: She's asleep now. You won't have to worry about her for the rest of the night.

If you were to guess what each of the three patients mentioned here were suffering from, what illnesses would you pick? If you'd rather not pick a specific illness, guess the seriousness of the illness and the probable prognosis. In small groups, arrive at some consensus for each patient—Ms. Ganon, Ms. Barnes, and Ms. Crandon. As a group, see if you can determine the clues in the conversation between the two nurses that led you to your theory about the seriousness of each patient's condition.

In the past, groups of nurses have agreed that Ms. Ganon and Ms. Barnes are probably postoperative, having undergone rather routine surgical procedures. Obviously, Ms. Barnes is almost fully recovered, and Ms. Ganon will probably be released soon.

They think Ms. Crandon, on the other hand, is probaly suffering from terminal cancer and has not long to live.

The nurses agreed that the apparent feelings and attitudes of the nurses revealed the condition of the patients. For example, Ms. Ganon may have been having pain, but it was manageable, and the nurses did not seem to have any great emotion about it. Nor did they refer to any feelings—besides pain—that Ms. Ganon might have. It seemed to them that this kind of cool professional discussion was more likely in the event of a relatively nonserious illness.

It was also clear that Ms. Barnes—though she was very vocal about how she felt—was in fairly good condition. For one thing, the nurses' disapproval and even dislike of her was evident, and most of the observers thought they would not be talking that way about her if she were seriously ill.

Mention by the nurses of Ms. Crandon revealed 1) reluctance to talk about her and some discomfort in doing so; 2) a patient so disturbed that the nurses wanted to increase medication *to reduce or extinguish her emotional responses,* rather than to deal with pain or with the illness itself; 3) an avoidance of the patient; 4) feelings of guilt about the relationship with the patient.

After you have finished your discussion and, perhaps, come to similar conclusions, here is some additional information. Actually, Ms. Ganon has had a myocardial infarction and is seriously ill. She is likely to die within the next week or so. How does your group now explain the conversational clues that led you to believe Ms. Ganon's prognosis was good? Is it possible that heart disease does not carry, *for you,* the same sense of despair and anxiety that cancer does? Do you, because of this, perceive an MI patient as less anxious and depressed than a cancer patient? Do you also feel more comfortable interacting with a heart patient than with a cancer patient, even though death is imminent for both of them? Does heart disease permit you more *hope* for recovery—even though there is no realistic basis for this hope—and so is more consistent with the traditional function of the nurse as one of healing and prolonging life?

Can you see yourself in the place of Ms. Ganon's nurse? Would your attitude be the same as the nurse's in the anecdote, or would it be different? Most people respond that it would probably be the same, that people with heart disease were easier to deal with than were people with terminal cancer. (Note they did not indicate they knew Ms. Ganon had "terminal" heart disease, although she died two days later.)

Before we leave this case study, here is another piece of information. Ms. Crandon was admitted to the hospital with a mild kidney dysfunction. There was never any question of cancer. If you were her nurse, describe how your behavior would be different from the behavior of the nurses in the story.

Actually, Ms. Crandon was a woman for whom a stay in the hospital— even for a minor illness—was in itself a very disturbing experience. She had three small children who had been distributed to relatives and friends, and the thought of their being separated made her feel very bad. She was a pleasant woman, quiet and uncomplaining, even though she was obviously unhappy. Having people around her to converse with and reassure her would have been helpful, but the nurses felt they could not afford to spend a lot of time with someone whose medical condition was under control—especially when there were so many other patients who needed care. But they liked her, felt sympathetic, and consequently a little guilty that they could not spend more time with her.

If your interpretation of the behavior was wrong, it was consistent with what usually does happen in the treatment of patients. Perhaps we need to look a little more closely into the real feelings of heart patients, for example. Maybe they need more help with their fears and anxieties than we think they do. Maybe, also, we should examine carefully every "reason" given for spending less time with patients dying of diseases like cancer. Does a diagnosis of inevitable death make the medical person reluctant to continue to give more than just medical care? Does he insulate himself behind his professional expertise as soon as he gives up hope of prolonging life, and become too busy to do more than make the patient "comfortable?" Does the patient dying of cancer suddenly become a medical case instead of a *living, needing* human being?

Discussion

An obvious question posed by the preceding exercises is this: In actual practice, is the professional functioning of the nurse severely circumscribed as soon as he learns the patient is dying? Is it possible, when gaining this knowledge, that he immediately begins to emphasize his strictly medical function, and slowly permits his social behavior to disappear?

(Social behaviors in this context might be identified as touching without a medical objective, demonstrating a feeling of comfort in interacting when no medical procedure is going on, extending a visit beyond the merely perfunctory, being clearly receptive to what the patient has to say and responding with obvious honesty.)

There is some evidence that this behavior does happen. It is not difficult to predict the possible causes:

1. A nurse, feeling more competent in the area of medical functioning and less competent in the social aspects of interaction with a person who is dying, may simply withdraw from social functioning and thus avoid the danger of making a mistake.
2. A nurse who is suddenly confronted with the inevitability of "failure" of his professional goal of healing the sick may insulate himself from his own feelings of frustration, anger, and despair by interposing his professional routines between himself and the patient who is triggering those feelings.
3. A nurse who wishes to protect himself from feelings of failure and sorrow may accept the admonitions from supervisors and teachers not to get emotionally involved with his patients because such involvement was unprofessional.
4. A nurse may recoil from the sudden awareness of her own mortality, and use her efficiency to control her fear.

Selected Bibliography

Books

Anthony, E. James, and Koupernik, Cyrille, eds. "The Child in his family." In *The impact of disease and death*. Vol. 2. New York: Wiley and Sons, 1973.

Anthony, Sylvia. *The child's discovery of death; a study in child psychology*, Harcourt Brace Jovanovich, Inc. 1940.

Becker, Ernest. *The denial of death*. New York: The Free Press, 1973.

Bermann, Eric. *Scapegoat; the impact of death-fear on an American family*. Ann Arbor: University of Michigan Press, 1973.

Blake, Robert R. *Attitudes toward death as a function of developmental stages*. Orange City, Iowa: Northwestern University, 1969. (Thesis)

Blum, R. H. et al. *The management of the doctor-patient relationship*, New York: McGraw-Hill, 1960.

Brim, Orville Gilbert, Jr., et al, eds. *Dying patient*. New York: Russell Sage Foundation, 1970.

Caring for the dying patient and his family; a model for medical education-medical center conferences. New York: Published for the Foundation of Thanatology by Health Sciences Publishing Corp., 1973.

Carson, William J. *Modes of coping with death concern*. Columbia: University of Missouri-Columbia, 1973. (Thesis)

Choron, Jacques. *Death and western thought*. New York: Collier Books, 1963.

Cook, Sarah, et. al. *Children and dying: an exploration and a selective professional bibliography*. New York: Health Sciences Publishing Corp., 1973.

Death education: preparation for living. Cambridge: Schenkman Publishing Co., 1971.

Dumont, Richard, and Foss, Dennis. *The American view of death: acceptance or denial?* Cambridge: Schenkman Publishing Co., 1972.

Feifel, H., ed. *The meaning of death*. New York: McGraw-Hill Book Co., 1959.

Flew, Antony Garrard Newton, ed. *Body, mind and death*. New York: The Macmillan Co., 1964.

Freud, Sigmund. *Civilization and its discontents*. London: Hogarth Press, 1933.

————. *Mourning and melancholia*. London: Hogarth Press, 1957.

————. "Thoughts for the times on war and death," *Collected papers*, Vol. 4, London: Hogarth Press, 1948.

————. *Totem and taboo*. New York: W. W. Norton and Co., Inc., 1952.

Fulton, Robert Lester. *Death and identity*. New York: Wiley, 1965.

Gatch, Milton. *Death: meaning and mortality in Christian thought and contemporary culture*. New York: Scabury Press, 1969.

Glaser, Barney G., and Strauss, Anselm L. *Awareness of dying*. Chicago: Aldine Publishing Co., 1965.

————. *Time for dying*. Chicago: Aldine Press, 1968.

Gordon, David C. *Overcoming the fear of death*. New York: Macmillan, 1970.

Gorer, Geoffrey. *Death, grief and mourning*. Garden City: Doubleday and Co., Inc., 1965.

Grollman, Earl A. *Explaining death to children*. Boston: Beacon Press, 1967.

Henderson, Joseph L. *The wisdom of the serpent; the myths of death, rebirth, and resurrection*. G. Braziller, 1963.

Hendin, David. *Death as a fact of life*. New York: Norton, 1973.

Hineman, Joseph H. *Counseling with the terminally ill: a clinical study*. Salt Lake City: University of Utah, 1971. (Thesis)

Hoblit, Pamela R. *An investigation of changes in anxiety level following consideration of death in four groups*. Baton Rouge: Louisiana State University and Agricultural and Mechanical College, 1972. (Thesis)

Jackson, Edgar Newman. *Telling a child about death*. Channel Press, 1965.

Kasmarik, Patricia E. *Attitude score changes toward death and dying in nursing students*. New York: Columbia University, 1974. (Thesis)

Kastenbaum, Robert J. "Loving, dying, and other gerontologic addenda." In *The psychology of adult development and aging*, edited by C.

Eisdorfer and M. P. Lawton. Washington, D.C.: American Psychological Association, 1973.

———, and Aisenberg, Ruth. *The Psychology of death.* New York: Springer Publishing Co., 1972.

———, and Weisman, A. D. "The Psychological autopsy as a research procedure in gerontology." In *Research planning and action for the elderly,* edited by D. P. Kent et. al. New York: Behavioral Publications, 1972.

Kavanaugh, Robert. *Facing death.* Los Angeles: Nash Publishing, 1973.

Kübler-Ross, Elizabeth. *On death and dying.* New York: Macmillan, 1969.

———. *Questions and answers on death and dying.* New York: Macmillan, 1974.

Kutscher, Austin H. Jr., and Kutscher, Austin H. *Bibliography of books on death, bereavement, loss and grief,* 1935-1968. New York: Health Sciences Publishing Corp. 1969.

Kutscher, Austin H. *Death and bereavement.* Springfield: Charles C. Thomas, 1969.

———, and Kutscher, Lillian G. *For the bereaved.* New York: F. Fell, 1971.

Lucas, Richard A. *A comparative study of measures of general anxiety and death anxiety among three medical groups including patient and wife.* Chapel Hill: University of North Carolina at Chapel Hill, 1972. (Thesis)

Marks, Elaine. *Simone de Beauvoir: encounters with death.* Rutgers University Press, 1973.

Melear, John D. *Children's conceptions of death.* Greeley: University of Northern Colorado, 1972. (Thesis)

Mills, Liston. *Perspectives on death.* Nashville: Abingdon Press, 1969.

Mitchell, Marjorie E. *The child's attitude to death.* London: Barrie and Rockliff in association with the Pemberton Publishing Co., 1966.

Mitford, Jessica. *The American way of death.* New York: Simon and Schuster Inc., 1963.

Munnichs, J. M. A. *Old age and finitude; a contribution to psychogerontology.* Basil, N.Y.: S. Karger, 1966.

Myler, Beatrice B. *Depression and death in the aged.* Boston: Boston University, 1967. (Thesis)

Neale, Robert E. *The art of dying.* New York: Harper and Row, 1973.

Nobel Conference, 8th Gustavus Adolphus College, 1972. *The end of life;* a discussion at the Nobel Conference, organized by Gustavus Adolphus College, St. Peter, Minnesota, 1972. Amsterdam: North-Holland Publishing Co., New York: Fleet Academic Editions, 1973.

Orwell, George. "How the poor die." In *Shooting an elephant.* Harcourt, Brace & World, Inc., 1950.

Pattison, E. M. *"Help in the dying process."* In: Arieti, S., ed. *American handbook of psychiatry. Vol. I. The Foundation of psychiatry.* New York: Basic Books, 1973.

Pearson, Leonard, ed. *Death and dying: current issues in the treatment of the dying person.* Cleveland: Case Western Reserve University Press, 1969.

Quint, Jeanne C. *The nurse and the dying patient.* New York: Macmillan, 1967.

Redick, Robert J. *Behavioral group counseling and death anxiety in student nurses.* Pittsburgh: University of Pittsburgh, 1974. (Thesis)

Reik, Theodor. *Curiosities of the self; illusions we have about ourselves.* Farrar, Straus and Giroux, 1965.

Ruitenbeek, Hendrik M. *The Interpretation of death.* J. Aronson, 1973.

Schneidman, Edwin S. *Death and the college student.* Behavioral Publications, 1972.

Schoenberg, Bernard, et al. *Loss and grief; psychological management in medical practice.* New York: Columbia University Press, 1970.

Scott, Frances, and Brewer, Ruth. *Confrontations of death; a book of readings and a suggested method of instruction.* Corvallis: Continuing Education Publications. Oregon State University, 1971.

Spinetta, John J. *Death anxiety in leukemic children.* Los Angeles: University of Southern California, 1972. (Thesis)

Sudnow, David. *Passing on; the social organization of dying.* Englewood Cliffs, N.J.: Prentice-Hall, 1967.

Symposium on death and attitudes toward death, University of Minnesota, 1972. *Death and attitudes toward death; proceedings.* Minneapolis: Bell Museum of Pathology, 1972.

Toynbee, Arnold, et al. *Man's concern with death.* McGraw-Hill, 1968.

Vernick, Joel J. *Selected bibliography on death and dying.* Washington, D.C.: U.S. National Institutes of Health, 1969.

Vernon, Glenn M. *Sociology of death; an analysis of death-related behavior.* New York: Ronald, 1970.

Walker, Kenneth M. *The circle of life: a search for an attitude to pain, disease, old age and death.* College Park, Md.: McGrath Publishing Co., 1970.

Warner, William Lloyd. *The living and the dead; a study of the symbolic life of Americans.* New Haven: Yale University Press, 1959.

Weisman, Avery D. *On dying and denying; a psychiatric study of terminality.* New York: Behavioral Publications, 1972.

Wesch, Jerry E. *Self-actualization and the fear of death.* Knoxville: University of Tennessee, 1970. (Thesis)

Zhiani-Rezai, Z. *Doctors and death.* Eugene: University of Oregon, 1968. (Thesis)

Periodicals

Aldrich, C. Knight. "The Dying Patient's Grief," *Journal of the American medical association*, 184, no. 5 (May 1963), pp. 329-331.

Annis, J. W. "The Dying patient." *Psychosomatics,* 10 (1969):289-292.

Ayd, Frank J., Jr. "What is death" *Medical counterpoint* (March 1974), 26-28.

Barton, David. "The Need for including instruction on death and dying in the medical curriculum." *Journal of medical education,* 47 (1972): 169-175.

————. "Teaching psychiatry in the context of dying and death." *American journal of psychiatry,* 130 (1973):1290-1291.

————, et al. "Death and dying: a course for medical students." *Journal of medical education,* 47 (1972):945-951.

Bascue, L. O., and Krieger, G. W. "Death as a counseling concern." *Personnel and guidance journal,* 52 (1974):587-592.

Berg, C. D. "Cognizance of the death taboo in counseling children." *School counselor,* 21 (1973):28-33.

Berg, David, and Daugherty, George. "Teaching about death." *Today's education,* 62 (March 1973):46-47.

Berman, Eric. "Death terror: observations of interaction patterns in an American family." *Omega,* 4 (1973):275-291.

Blazer, John A. "The Relationship between meaning in life and fear of death." *Psychology,* 10 (1973):33-34.

Branscomb, Allan, and Branscomb, Elbert. "Sharing: a death research information exchange." *Omega,* 4 (1973):243-249.

Bulger, Roger. "The Dying patient and his doctor." *Harvard medical alumni bulletin,* 34, no. 3 (1960), pp. 23-25, 53-57.

Bynum, Jack. "Social status and rites of passage: the social context of death." *Omega,* 4 (1973):323-332.

Cappon, Daniel. "Attitudes on death." *Omega,* 1 (1970):103-108.

Chasin, B. "Neglected variables in the study of death attitudes." *Sociological quarterly,* 12 (1971):107-113.

Cramond, W. A. "Psychotherapy of the dying patient." *British medical journal,* 3 (1970):389-393.

Crase, D. R., and Crase, D. "Live issues surrounding death education." *Journal of school health,* 44 (1974):70-73.

Durlak, Joseph. "Relationship between individual attitudes toward life and death." *Journal of consulting and clinical psychology,* 38 (1972): 463.

Feifel, Herman. "Attitudes toward death: a psychological perspective." *Journal of consulting and clinical psychology,* 33 (1969):292-295.

Fisher, Gary. "Death, identity and creativity." *Omega,* 2 (1971):303-306.

———. "Psychotherapy for the dying: principles and illustrative cases with special references to the use of LSD." *Omega,* 1 (1970):3-15.

Fontenot, Christine. "The subject nobody teaches." *English journal,* 63 (1974):62-63.

Friedman, Henry J. "Physician management of dying patients: an exploration." *Psychiatry in medicine,* 1 (1970):295-305.

Fulton, Robert, and Fulton, Julie. "A Psychosocial aspect of terminal care:" anticipatory grief, *Omega,* 2 (1971):91-100.

Group for the Advancement of Psychiatry. "The Right to die: decision and decision makers." *GAP Report,* 8 (1973):667-751.

Guthrie, George P. "The Meaning of death." *Omega,* 2 (1971):299-302.

Gutmann, D. "The Premature gerontocracy: themes of aging and death in the youth culture." *Social research,* 39 (1972):416-448.

Hertzberg, Leonard. "Cancer and the dying patient." *American journal of psychiatry,* 128 (1972):806-810.

Hinton, John. "Assessing the views of the dying." *Social science and medicine,* 5 (1971):37-43.

Kahana, Boaz, and Kahana, Eva. "Attitudes of young men and women toward awareness of death." *Omega,* 3 (1972):37-44.

Kastenbaum, Robert. "The Mental health specialist and the American 'death system'." *Psychiatric opinion,* 9 (1972):28-37.

———. "On the future of death: some images and options." *Omega,* 3 (1972):306-318.

———, and Koenig, Ronald. "Dying, death and lethal behavior: an experience in community education." *Omega,* 1 (1970):29-36.

Kikuchi, June. "A Leukemic adolescent's verbalization about dying." *Maternal-child nursing journal,* 1 (1972):259-264.

Kimsey, Larry R., et al. "Death, dying and denial in the aged." *American journal of psychiatry,* 129 (1972):161-166.

Koestenbaum, Peter. "The Vitality of death." *Omega,* 2 (1971):253-271.

Koocher, Gerald P. "Childhood, death and cognitive development." *Developmental psychology,* 9 (1973):369-375.

Krahn, John H. "Pervasive death: an avoided concept." *Educational leadership,* 31 (1973):18-20.

Kron, Joan. "Learning to live with death." *Omega,* 5 (1974):5-24.

Krupp, G. "Maladaptive reactions to the death of a family member." *Social casework,* 53 (1972):425-434.

Kübler-Ross, Elizabeth. "The Care of the dying: whose job is it?" *Psychiatry in medicine,* 1 (1970):103-107.

———. "Facing up to death; terminally ill patients." *Today's education,* January 1972, 61:30-32.

Leviton, Dan. "A Course on death education and suicide prevention:

implications for health education." *American college health association journal*, 49 (1971):217-220.

Levy, Norman B. "Fatal illness: should the patient be told?" *Medical insight*, November 1973, 20-23.

Liston, Edward. "Education on death and dying: a survey of American medical schools." *Journal of medical education*, 48 (1973):577-578.

Lucente, Frank. "Thanatology, a study of 100 deaths on an otolarngology service." *Omega*, 3 (1972):211-216.

McLure, John. "Death education." *Phi delta kappan*, 55 (1974):483-485.

McMahon, J. D. "Death education: an independent study unit." *Journal of school health*, 43 (1973):526-527.

Marcovitz, Eli. "What is the meaning of death to the dying person and his survivors?" *Omega*, 4 (1973):13-25.

Meyerson, Henry. "The Psychology of the dying patient." *Osteopathic annals*, March 1974, 51-56.

Miller, Jill. "Children's reactions to the death of a parent: a review of the psychoanalytic literature." *American psychoanalytic association journal*, 19 (1971):697-719.

Moore, Joan. "The Death culture of Mexico and Mexican-Americans." *Omega*, 1 (1970):271-291.

Olin, Harry. "A proposed model to teach medical students the care of the dying patient." *Journal of medical education*, 47 (1972):564-576.

Parkin, Michael. "A proposal for the development of crisis counseling services related to dying, death, grief and mourning." *Crisis intervention*, 4 (1972):121-125.

Pattison, E. Mansell. "Psychosocial predictors of death prognosis." *Omega*, 5 (1974):145-160.

Pine, Vanderlyn. "Social organization and death." *Omega*, 3 (1972):149-153.

Quint, Jeanne C. "The Dying patient: A difficult nursing problem." *Nursing clinics of North America*, December 1967.

Rakoff, V. M. "Psychiatric aspects of death in America." *Social research*, 39 (1972):515-527.

Roose, Lawrence. "The Dying patient." *International journal of psychoanalysis*, 50 (1969):385-395.

Sabatini, Paul, and Kastenbaum, Robert. "The Do-it-yourself death certificate as a research technique." *Life threatening behavior*, 3 (1973):20-32.

Saul, Sidney, and Saul, Shura. "Old people talk about death." *Omega*, 4 (1973):27-35.

Schrank, J. "Death; guide to books and audio-visual aids." *Media and methods*, 7 (1971):32-54.

Scott, Byron T. "Physicians' attitude survey." *Medical opinion*, 3 (1974):32-34.

Seiden, Richard H. "We're driving young blacks to suicide." *Psychology today,* 4 August 1970:24-28.

Selvey, Carole. "Concerns about death in relation to sex, dependency, guilt about hostility and feelings of powerlessness." *Omega,* 4 (1973): 209-219.

Share, Lynda. "Family communication in the crisis of a child's fatal illness: a literature review and analysis." *Omega,* 3 (1972):187-201.

Shneidman, Edwin S. "Death questionnaire." *Psychology today,* 4 August 1970, 67-72.

———. "The enemy." *Psychology today,* August 1970, 37-41, 62-66.

———. "On the deromanticization of death." *American journal of psychotherapy,* 25 (1971):4-17.

———. "You and death." *Psychology today,* 5, June 1971, 43-45, 74-80.

Siggins, L. D. "Mourning: a critical survey of the literature." *International journal of psychiatry,* 3 (1967):418-432.

Solnit, Albert J., and Green, Morris. "Psychologic Considerations in the Management of Deaths on Pediatric Hospital Services." *Pediatrics,* 24, no. 1 (1959):106-112.

Somerville, R. M. "Death education as part of family life education: using imaginative literature for insights into family crisis." *Family coordinator,* 20 (1971):223-224.

Stephenson, Carolan. "Coping with death." *Southwestern sociological association,* 49th annual meeting papers, 1974.

Templer, D. I. "Construction and validation of death anxiety scale." *Journal of general psychology,* 82 (1970):176-177.

Vernon, Glenn M. "Changing interpretations of death." *Southern sociological society,* 34th annual meeting papers, 1971.

Vernon, Glenn. "Death control." *Omega,* 3 (1972): 131-138.

Vollman, Rita, et al. "The reaction of family systems to sudden and unexpected death." *Omega,* 2 (1971):101-106.

Wahl, Charles. "Helping the dying patient and his family." *Journal of pastoral care,* 26 (1972):93-98.

West, Norman. "The psychology of death in geriatrics." *American geriatrics society journal,* 20 (1972):340-342.

Wheeler, Allan L. "The dying person: a deviant in the medical subculture." *Southern sociological society,* 37th annual meeting papers, 1974.

White, Douglas. "An undergraduate course in death." *Omega,* 1 (1970): 167-174.

Wise, Doreen. "Learning about dying." *Nursing outlook,* 22 (1974):42-44.

Zazzaro, Joanne. "Death be not distorted." *Nation's schools,* 91 (1973):39-42, 102.

Index